Mometrix
TEST PREPARATION

EMT
Intermediate 99 Exam Secrets Study Guide

NREMT is a registered trademark of National Registry of Emergency Medical Technicians, which is not affiliated with Mometrix Test Preparation and does not endorse this product.

Dear Future Exam Success Story

First of all, **THANK YOU** for purchasing Mometrix study materials!

Second, congratulations! You are one of the few determined test-takers who are committed to doing whatever it takes to excel on your exam. **You have come to the right place.** We developed these study materials with one goal in mind: to deliver you the information you need in a format that's concise and easy to use.

In addition to optimizing your guide for the content of the test, we've outlined our recommended steps for breaking down the preparation process into small, attainable goals so you can make sure you stay on track.

We've also analyzed the entire test-taking process, identifying the most common pitfalls and showing how you can overcome them and be ready for any curveball the test throws you.

Standardized testing is one of the biggest obstacles on your road to success, which only increases the importance of doing well in the high-pressure, high-stakes environment of test day. Your results on this test could have a significant impact on your future, and this guide provides the information and practical advice to help you achieve your full potential on test day.

Your success is our success

We would love to hear from you! If you would like to share the story of your exam success or if you have any questions or comments in regard to our products, please contact us at **800-673-8175** or **support@mometrix.com**.

Thanks again for your business and we wish you continued success!

Sincerely,
The Mometrix Test Preparation Team

Need more help? Check out our flashcards at:
http://MometrixFlashcards.com/EMT

Copyright © 2026 by Mometrix Media LLC. All rights reserved.
Written and edited by the Mometrix Exam Secrets Test Prep Team
Printed in the United States of America

Table of Contents

Introduction	1
Secret Key #1 – Plan Big, Study Small	2
Secret Key #2 – Make Your Studying Count	3
Secret Key #3 – Practice the Right Way	4
Secret Key #4 – Pace Yourself	6
Secret Key #5 – Have a Plan for Guessing	7
Test-Taking Strategies	10
Preparatory	15
Anatomy and Physiology	35
Medical Terminology	36
Pathophysiology	37
Life Span Development	39
Public Health	40
Pharmacology	41
Airway Management, Respirations and Artificial Ventilation	43
Assessment	51
Medicine	55
Shock and Resuscitation	84
Trauma	88
Special Patient Populations	112
EMS Operations	122
EMT Practice Test	137
Answer Key and Explanations	156
Special Report: Difficult Clients	169
Special Report: Guidelines for Standard Precautions	170
Special Report: Basic Review of Types of Fractures	171
CPR Guidelines for Professional Rescuers	172
Online Resources	173

Introduction

Thank you for purchasing this resource! You have made the choice to prepare yourself for a test that could have a huge impact on your future, and this guide is designed to help you be fully ready for test day. Obviously, it's important to have a solid understanding of the test material, but you also need to be prepared for the unique environment and stressors of the test, so that you can perform to the best of your abilities.

For this purpose, the first section that appears in this guide is the **Secret Keys**. We've devoted countless hours to meticulously researching what works and what doesn't, and we've boiled down our findings to the five most impactful steps you can take to improve your performance on the test. We start at the beginning with study planning and move through the preparation process, all the way to the testing strategies that will help you get the most out of what you know when you're finally sitting in front of the test.

We recommend that you start preparing for your test as far in advance as possible. However, if you've bought this guide as a last-minute study resource and only have a few days before your test, we recommend that you skip over the first two Secret Keys since they address a long-term study plan.

If you struggle with **test anxiety**, we strongly encourage you to check out our recommendations for how you can overcome it. Test anxiety is a formidable foe, but it can be beaten, and we want to make sure you have the tools you need to defeat it.

Secret Key #1 – Plan Big, Study Small

There's a lot riding on your performance. If you want to ace this test, you're going to need to keep your skills sharp and the material fresh in your mind. You need a plan that lets you review everything you need to know while still fitting in your schedule. We'll break this strategy down into three categories.

Information Organization

Start with the information you already have: the official test outline. From this, you can make a complete list of all the concepts you need to cover before the test. Organize these concepts into groups that can be studied together, and create a list of any related vocabulary you need to learn so you can brush up on any difficult terms. You'll want to keep this vocabulary list handy once you actually start studying since you may need to add to it along the way.

Time Management

Once you have your set of study concepts, decide how to spread them out over the time you have left before the test. Break your study plan into small, clear goals so you have a manageable task for each day and know exactly what you're doing. Then just focus on one small step at a time. When you manage your time this way, you don't need to spend hours at a time studying. Studying a small block of content for a short period each day helps you retain information better and avoid stressing over how much you have left to do. You can relax knowing that you have a plan to cover everything in time. In order for this strategy to be effective though, you have to start studying early and stick to your schedule. Avoid the exhaustion and futility that comes from last-minute cramming!

Study Environment

The environment you study in has a big impact on your learning. Studying in a coffee shop, while probably more enjoyable, is not likely to be as fruitful as studying in a quiet room. It's important to keep distractions to a minimum. You're only planning to study for a short block of time, so make the most of it. Don't pause to check your phone or get up to find a snack. It's also important to **avoid multitasking**. Research has consistently shown that multitasking will make your studying dramatically less effective. Your study area should also be comfortable and well-lit so you don't have the distraction of straining your eyes or sitting on an uncomfortable chair.

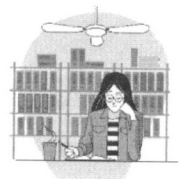

The time of day you study is also important. You want to be rested and alert. Don't wait until just before bedtime. Study when you'll be most likely to comprehend and remember. Even better, if you know what time of day your test will be, set that time aside for study. That way your brain will be used to working on that subject at that specific time and you'll have a better chance of recalling information.

Finally, it can be helpful to team up with others who are studying for the same test. Your actual studying should be done in as isolated an environment as possible, but the work of organizing the information and setting up the study plan can be divided up. In between study sessions, you can discuss with your teammates the concepts that you're all studying and quiz each other on the details. Just be sure that your teammates are as serious about the test as you are. If you find that your study time is being replaced with social time, you might need to find a new team.

Secret Key #2 – Make Your Studying Count

You're devoting a lot of time and effort to preparing for this test, so you want to be absolutely certain it will pay off. This means doing more than just reading the content and hoping you can remember it on test day. It's important to make every minute of study count. There are two main areas you can focus on to make your studying count.

Retention

It doesn't matter how much time you study if you can't remember the material. You need to make sure you are retaining the concepts. To check your retention of the information you're learning, try recalling it at later times with minimal prompting. Try carrying around flashcards and glance at one or two from time to time or ask a friend who's also studying for the test to quiz you.

To enhance your retention, look for ways to put the information into practice so that you can apply it rather than simply recalling it. If you're using the information in practical ways, it will be much easier to remember. Similarly, it helps to solidify a concept in your mind if you're not only reading it to yourself but also explaining it to someone else. Ask a friend to let you teach them about a concept you're a little shaky on (or speak aloud to an imaginary audience if necessary). As you try to summarize, define, give examples, and answer your friend's questions, you'll understand the concepts better and they will stay with you longer. Finally, step back for a big picture view and ask yourself how each piece of information fits with the whole subject. When you link the different concepts together and see them working together as a whole, it's easier to remember the individual components.

Finally, practice showing your work on any multi-step problems, even if you're just studying. Writing out each step you take to solve a problem will help solidify the process in your mind, and you'll be more likely to remember it during the test.

Modality

Modality simply refers to the means or method by which you study. Choosing a study modality that fits your own individual learning style is crucial. No two people learn best in exactly the same way, so it's important to know your strengths and use them to your advantage.

For example, if you learn best by visualization, focus on visualizing a concept in your mind and draw an image or a diagram. Try color-coding your notes, illustrating them, or creating symbols that will trigger your mind to recall a learned concept. If you learn best by hearing or discussing information, find a study partner who learns the same way or read aloud to yourself. Think about how to put the information in your own words. Imagine that you are giving a lecture on the topic and record yourself so you can listen to it later.

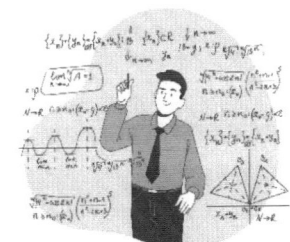

For any learning style, flashcards can be helpful. Organize the information so you can take advantage of spare moments to review. Underline key words or phrases. Use different colors for different categories. Mnemonic devices (such as creating a short list in which every item starts with the same letter) can also help with retention. Find what works best for you and use it to store the information in your mind most effectively and easily.

Secret Key #3 – Practice the Right Way

Your success on test day depends not only on how many hours you put into preparing, but also on whether you prepared the right way. It's good to check along the way to see if your studying is paying off. One of the most effective ways to do this is by taking practice tests to evaluate your progress. Practice tests are useful because they show exactly where you need to improve. Every time you take a practice test, pay special attention to these three groups of questions:

- The questions you got wrong
- The questions you had to guess on, even if you guessed right
- The questions you found difficult or slow to work through

This will show you exactly what your weak areas are, and where you need to devote more study time. Ask yourself why each of these questions gave you trouble. Was it because you didn't understand the material? Was it because you didn't remember the vocabulary? Do you need more repetitions on this type of question to build speed and confidence? Dig into those questions and figure out how you can strengthen your weak areas as you go back to review the material.

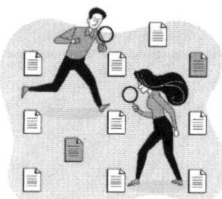
Additionally, many practice tests have a section explaining the answer choices. It can be tempting to read the explanation and think that you now have a good understanding of the concept. However, an explanation likely only covers part of the question's broader context. Even if the explanation makes perfect sense, **go back and investigate** every concept related to the question until you're positive you have a thorough understanding.

As you go along, keep in mind that the practice test is just that: practice. Memorizing these questions and answers will not be very helpful on the actual test because it is unlikely to have any of the same exact questions. If you only know the right answers to the sample questions, you won't be prepared for the real thing. **Study the concepts** until you understand them fully, and then you'll be able to answer any question that shows up on the test.

It's important to wait on the practice tests until you're ready. If you take a test on your first day of study, you may be overwhelmed by the amount of material covered and how much you need to learn. Work up to it gradually.

On test day, you'll need to be prepared for answering questions, managing your time, and using the test-taking strategies you've learned. It's a lot to balance, like a mental marathon that will have a big impact on your future. Like training for a marathon, you'll need to start slowly and work your way up. When test day arrives, you'll be ready.

Start with the strategies you've read in the first two Secret Keys—plan your course and study in the way that works best for you. If you have time, consider using multiple study resources to get different approaches to the same concepts. It can be helpful to see difficult concepts from more than one angle. Then find a good source for practice tests. Many times, the test website will suggest potential study resources or provide sample tests.

Practice Test Strategy

If you're able to find at least three practice tests, we recommend this strategy:

Untimed and Open-Book Practice

Take the first test with no time constraints and with your notes and study guide handy. Take your time and focus on applying the strategies you've learned.

Timed and Open-Book Practice

Take the second practice test open-book as well, but set a timer and practice pacing yourself to finish in time.

Timed and Closed-Book Practice

Take any other practice tests as if it were test day. Set a timer and put away your study materials. Sit at a table or desk in a quiet room, imagine yourself at the testing center, and answer questions as quickly and accurately as possible.

Keep repeating timed and closed-book tests on a regular basis until you run out of practice tests or it's time for the actual test. Your mind will be ready for the schedule and stress of test day, and you'll be able to focus on recalling the material you've learned.

Secret Key #4 – Pace Yourself

Once you're fully prepared for the material on the test, your biggest challenge on test day will be managing your time. Just knowing that the clock is ticking can make you panic even if you have plenty of time left. Work on pacing yourself so you can build confidence against the time constraints of the exam. Pacing is a difficult skill to master, especially in a high-pressure environment, so **practice is vital**.

Set time expectations for your pace based on how much time is available. For example, if a section has 60 questions and the time limit is 30 minutes, you know you have to average 30 seconds or less per question in order to answer them all. Although 30 seconds is the hard limit, set 25 seconds per question as your goal, so you reserve extra time to spend on harder questions. When you budget extra time for the harder questions, you no longer have any reason to stress when those questions take longer to answer.

Don't let this time expectation distract you from working through the test at a calm, steady pace, but keep it in mind so you don't spend too much time on any one question. Recognize that taking extra time on one question you don't understand may keep you from answering two that you do understand later in the test. If your time limit for a question is up and you're still not sure of the answer, mark it and move on, and come back to it later if the time and the test format allow. If the testing format doesn't allow you to return to earlier questions, just make an educated guess; then put it out of your mind and move on.

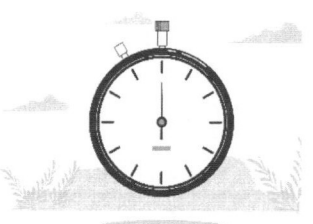

On the easier questions, be careful not to rush. It may seem wise to hurry through them so you have more time for the challenging ones, but it's not worth missing one if you know the concept and just didn't take the time to read the question fully. Work efficiently but make sure you understand the question and have looked at all of the answer choices, since more than one may seem right at first.

Even if you're paying attention to the time, you may find yourself a little behind at some point. You should speed up to get back on track, but do so wisely. Don't panic; just take a few seconds less on each question until you're caught up. Don't guess without thinking, but do look through the answer choices and eliminate any you know are wrong. If you can get down to two choices, it is often worthwhile to guess from those. Once you've chosen an answer, move on and don't dwell on any that you skipped or had to hurry through. If a question was taking too long, chances are it was one of the harder ones, so you weren't as likely to get it right anyway.

On the other hand, if you find yourself getting ahead of schedule, it may be beneficial to slow down a little. The more quickly you work, the more likely you are to make a careless mistake that will affect your score. You've budgeted time for each question, so don't be afraid to spend that time. Practice an efficient but careful pace to get the most out of the time you have.

Secret Key #5 – Have a Plan for Guessing

When you're taking the test, you may find yourself stuck on a question. Some of the answer choices seem better than others, but you don't see the one answer choice that is obviously correct. What do you do?

The scenario described above is very common, yet most test takers have not effectively prepared for it. Developing and practicing a plan for guessing may be one of the single most effective uses of your time as you get ready for the exam.

In developing your plan for guessing, there are three questions to address:

- When should you start the guessing process?
- How should you narrow down the choices?
- Which answer should you choose?

When to Start the Guessing Process

Unless your plan for guessing is to select C every time (which, despite its merits, is not what we recommend), you need to leave yourself enough time to apply your answer elimination strategies. Since you have a limited amount of time for each question, that means that if you're going to give yourself the best shot at guessing correctly, you have to decide quickly whether or not you will guess.

Of course, the best-case scenario is that you don't have to guess at all, so first, see if you can answer the question based on your knowledge of the subject and basic reasoning skills. Focus on the key words in the question and try to jog your memory of related topics. Give yourself a chance to bring the knowledge to mind, but once you realize that you don't have (or you can't access) the knowledge you need to answer the question, it's time to start the guessing process.

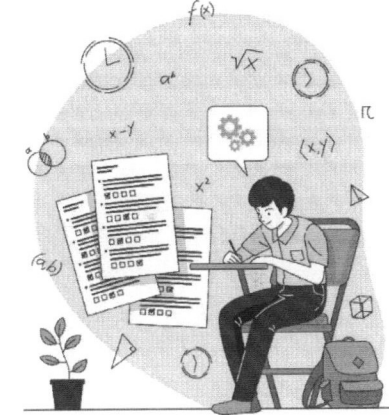

It's almost always better to start the guessing process too early than too late. It only takes a few seconds to remember something and answer the question from knowledge. Carefully eliminating wrong answer choices takes longer. Plus, going through the process of eliminating answer choices can actually help jog your memory.

Summary: Start the guessing process as soon as you decide that you can't answer the question based on your knowledge.

How to Narrow Down the Choices

The next chapter in this book (**Test-Taking Strategies**) includes a wide range of strategies for how to approach questions and how to look for answer choices to eliminate. You will definitely want to read those carefully, practice them, and figure out which ones work best for you. Here though, we're going to address a mindset rather than a particular strategy.

Your odds of guessing an answer correctly depend on how many options you are choosing from.

Number of options left	5	4	3	2	1
Odds of guessing correctly	20%	25%	33%	50%	100%

You can see from this chart just how valuable it is to be able to eliminate incorrect answers and make an educated guess, but there are two things that many test takers do that cause them to miss out on the benefits of guessing:

- Accidentally eliminating the correct answer
- Selecting an answer based on an impression

We'll look at the first one here, and the second one in the next section.

To avoid accidentally eliminating the correct answer, we recommend a thought exercise called **the $5 challenge**. In this challenge, you only eliminate an answer choice from contention if you are willing to bet $5 on it being wrong. Why $5? Five dollars is a small but not insignificant amount of money. It's an amount you could afford to lose but wouldn't want to throw away. And while losing $5 once might not hurt too much, doing it twenty times will set you back $100. In the same way, each small decision you make—eliminating a choice here, guessing on a question there—won't by itself impact your score very much, but when you put them all together, they can make a big difference. By holding each answer choice elimination decision to a higher standard, you can reduce the risk of accidentally eliminating the correct answer.

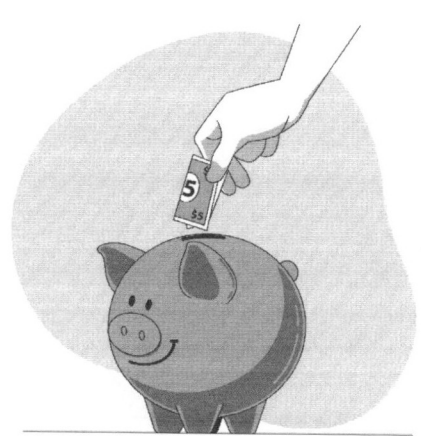

The $5 challenge can also be applied in a positive sense: If you are willing to bet $5 that an answer choice *is* correct, go ahead and mark it as correct.

Summary: Only eliminate an answer choice if you are willing to bet $5 that it is wrong.

Which Answer to Choose

You're taking the test. You've run into a hard question and decided you'll have to guess. You've eliminated all the answer choices you're willing to bet $5 on. Now you have to pick an answer. Why do we even need to talk about this? Why can't you just pick whichever one you feel like when the time comes?

The answer to these questions is that if you don't come into the test with a plan, you'll rely on your impression to select an answer choice, and if you do that, you risk falling into a trap. The test writers know that everyone who takes their test will be guessing on some of the questions, so they intentionally write wrong answer choices to seem plausible. You still have to pick an answer though, and if the wrong answer choices are designed to look right, how can you ever be sure that you're not falling for their trap? The best solution we've found to this dilemma is to take the decision out of your hands entirely. Here is the process we recommend:

Once you've eliminated any choices that you are confident (willing to bet $5) are wrong, select the first remaining choice as your answer.

Whether you choose to select the first remaining choice, the second, or the last, the important thing is that you use some preselected standard. Using this approach guarantees that you will not be enticed into selecting an answer choice that looks right, because you are not basing your decision on how the answer choices look.

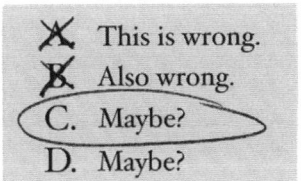

This is not meant to make you question your knowledge. Instead, it is to help you recognize the difference between your knowledge and your impressions. There's a huge difference between thinking an answer is right because of what you know, and thinking an answer is right because it looks or sounds like it should be right.

Summary: To ensure that your selection is appropriately random, make a predetermined selection from among all answer choices you have not eliminated.

Test-Taking Strategies

This section contains a list of test-taking strategies that you may find helpful as you work through the test. By taking what you know and applying logical thought, you can maximize your chances of answering any question correctly!

It is very important to realize that every question is different and every person is different: no single strategy will work on every question, and no single strategy will work for every person. That's why we've included all of them here, so you can try them out and determine which ones work best for different types of questions and which ones work best for you.

Question Strategies

ⓥ READ CAREFULLY

Read the question and the answer choices carefully. Don't miss the question because you misread the terms. You have plenty of time to read each question thoroughly and make sure you understand what is being asked. Yet a happy medium must be attained, so don't waste too much time. You must read carefully and efficiently.

ⓥ CONTEXTUAL CLUES

Look for contextual clues. If the question includes a word you are not familiar with, look at the immediate context for some indication of what the word might mean. Contextual clues can often give you all the information you need to decipher the meaning of an unfamiliar word. Even if you can't determine the meaning, you may be able to narrow down the possibilities enough to make a solid guess at the answer to the question.

ⓥ PREFIXES

If you're having trouble with a word in the question or answer choices, try dissecting it. Take advantage of every clue that the word might include. Prefixes can be a huge help. Usually, they allow you to determine a basic meaning. *Pre-* means before, *post-* means after, *pro-* is positive, *de-* is negative. From prefixes, you can get an idea of the general meaning of the word and try to put it into context.

ⓥ HEDGE WORDS

Watch out for critical hedge words, such as *likely, may, can, often, almost, mostly, usually, generally, rarely,* and *sometimes*. Question writers insert these hedge phrases to cover every possibility. Often an answer choice will be wrong simply because it leaves no room for exception. Be on guard for answer choices that have definitive words such as *exactly* and *always*.

ⓥ SWITCHBACK WORDS

Stay alert for *switchbacks*. These are the words and phrases frequently used to alert you to shifts in thought. The most common switchback words are *but, although,* and *however*. Others include *nevertheless, on the other hand, even though, while, in spite of, despite,* and *regardless of*. Switchback words are important to catch because they can change the direction of the question or an answer choice.

ⓥ FACE VALUE

When in doubt, use common sense. Accept the situation in the problem at face value. Don't read too much into it. These problems will not require you to make wild assumptions. If you have to go beyond creativity and warp time or space in order to have an answer choice fit the question, then you should move on and consider the other answer choices. These are normal problems rooted in reality. The applicable relationship or explanation may not be readily apparent, but it is there for you to figure out. Use your common sense to interpret anything that isn't clear.

Answer Choice Strategies

✓ Answer Selection
The most thorough way to pick an answer choice is to identify and eliminate wrong answers until only one is left, then confirm it is the correct answer. Sometimes an answer choice may immediately seem right, but be careful. The test writers will usually put more than one reasonable answer choice on each question, so take a second to read all of them and make sure that the other choices are not equally obvious. As long as you have time left, it is better to read every answer choice than to pick the first one that looks right without checking the others.

✓ Answer Choice Families
An answer choice family consists of two (in rare cases, three) answer choices that are very similar in construction and cannot all be true at the same time. If you see two answer choices that are direct opposites or parallels, one of them is usually the correct answer. For instance, if one answer choice says that quantity x increases and another either says that quantity x decreases (opposite) or says that quantity y increases (parallel), then those answer choices would fall into the same family. An answer choice that doesn't match the construction of the answer choice family is more likely to be incorrect. Most questions will not have answer choice families, but when they do appear, you should be prepared to recognize them.

✓ Eliminate Answers
Eliminate answer choices as soon as you realize they are wrong, but make sure you consider all possibilities. If you are eliminating answer choices and realize that the last one you are left with is also wrong, don't panic. Start over and consider each choice again. There may be something you missed the first time that you will realize on the second pass.

✓ Avoid Fact Traps
Don't be distracted by an answer choice that is factually true but doesn't answer the question. You are looking for the choice that answers the question. Stay focused on what the question is asking for so you don't accidentally pick an answer that is true but incorrect. Always go back to the question and make sure the answer choice you've selected actually answers the question and is not merely a true statement.

✓ Extreme Statements
In general, you should avoid answers that put forth extreme actions as standard practice or proclaim controversial ideas as established fact. An answer choice that states the "process should be used in certain situations, if…" is much more likely to be correct than one that states the "process should be discontinued completely." The first is a calm rational statement and doesn't even make a definitive, uncompromising stance, using a hedge word *if* to provide wiggle room, whereas the second choice is far more extreme.

✓ Benchmark
As you read through the answer choices and you come across one that seems to answer the question well, mentally select that answer choice. This is not your final answer, but it's the one that will help you evaluate the other answer choices. The one that you selected is your benchmark or standard for judging each of the other answer choices. Every other answer choice must be compared to your benchmark. That choice is correct until proven otherwise by another answer choice beating it. If you find a better answer, then that one becomes your new benchmark. Once you've decided that no other choice answers the question as well as your benchmark, you have your final answer.

⊘ Predict the Answer

Before you even start looking at the answer choices, it is often best to try to predict the answer. When you come up with the answer on your own, it is easier to avoid distractions and traps because you will know exactly what to look for. The right answer choice is unlikely to be word-for-word what you came up with, but it should be a close match. Even if you are confident that you have the right answer, you should still take the time to read each option before moving on.

General Strategies

⊘ Tough Questions

If you are stumped on a problem or it appears too hard or too difficult, don't waste time. Move on! Remember though, if you can quickly check for obviously incorrect answer choices, your chances of guessing correctly are greatly improved. Before you completely give up, at least try to knock out a couple of possible answers. Eliminate what you can and then guess at the remaining answer choices before moving on.

⊘ Check Your Work

Since you will probably not know every term listed and the answer to every question, it is important that you get credit for the ones that you do know. Don't miss any questions through careless mistakes. If at all possible, try to take a second to look back over your answer selection and make sure you've selected the correct answer choice and haven't made a costly careless mistake (such as marking an answer choice that you didn't mean to mark). This quick double check should more than pay for itself in caught mistakes for the time it costs.

⊘ Pace Yourself

It's easy to be overwhelmed when you're looking at a page full of questions; your mind is confused and full of random thoughts, and the clock is ticking down faster than you would like. Calm down and maintain the pace that you have set for yourself. Especially as you get down to the last few minutes of the test, don't let the small numbers on the clock make you panic. As long as you are on track by monitoring your pace, you are guaranteed to have time for each question.

⊘ Don't Rush

It is very easy to make errors when you are in a hurry. Maintaining a fast pace in answering questions is pointless if it makes you miss questions that you would have gotten right otherwise. Test writers like to include distracting information and wrong answers that seem right. Taking a little extra time to avoid careless mistakes can make all the difference in your test score. Find a pace that allows you to be confident in the answers that you select.

⊘ Keep Moving

Panicking will not help you pass the test, so do your best to stay calm and keep moving. Taking deep breaths and going through the answer elimination steps you practiced can help to break through a stress barrier and keep your pace.

Final Notes

The combination of a solid foundation of content knowledge and the confidence that comes from practicing your plan for applying that knowledge is the key to maximizing your performance on test day. As your foundation of content knowledge is built up and strengthened, you'll find that the strategies included in this chapter become more and more effective in helping you quickly sift through the distractions and traps of the test to isolate the correct answer.

Now that you're preparing to move forward into the test content chapters of this book, be sure to keep your goal in mind. As you read, think about how you will be able to apply this information on the test. If you've already seen sample questions for the test and you have an idea of the question format and style, try to come up with questions of your own that you can answer based on what you're reading. This will give you valuable practice applying your knowledge in the same ways you can expect to on test day.

Good luck and good studying!

Preparatory

EMS Systems

The National Highway Traffic Safety Administration (NHTSA) is the lead agency for coordinating and promoting evidence-based emergency medical services (EMS) (fire based, third service, and hospital based) and the 9-1-1 system. The public safety answering point (PSAP) is the designated call-receiving site that directs calls to the appropriate emergency services. Each state defines the scope of practice, licensure, and credentialing for prehospital personnel and sets education standards based on national EMS standards. The advanced emergency medical technician (AEMT) is expected to maintain certification through maintenance of skills and continuing education and should exhibit professional behavior, including working with integrity and empathy, being an effective member of a team, showing respect and tact, maintaining a professional appearance, communicating effectively, and advocating for patients. The AEMT must be alert to patient safety and recognize that most errors result from skills-based, rules-based, and knowledge-based failures. Error reduction requires the use of decision aids and protocols, asking for assistance when appropriate, questioning assumptions, and debriefing calls.

Patient Safety and High-Risk Situations

Up to 98,000 patients die each year because of medical errors. Patients are especially at risk of further injury or death in high-risk situations and activities such as the following:

- Hand-off: A standard procedure, such as SBAR, should be used, as follows:
    - (S) Situation: Overview of current situation and important issues.
    - (B) Background: Important history and issues leading to current situation.
    - Assessment: Summary of important facts and condition.
    - (R) Recommendation: Actions needed.
- Communications: Problems may result in delayed or inadequate care, wrong address, or wrong destination.
- Dropping: Patients can be easily dropped if the gurney isn't positioned properly or if too few personnel are involved in transport.
- Ambulance crashes: Unnecessary speeding and failing to stop at intersections are the most common causes of ambulance crashes.
- Inadequate spinal immobilization: If unsure, it's always best to immobilize.
- Medication errors: Administration of wrong medication, wrong mode of administration, and wrong dosage.

Roles and Responsibilities of EMS Personnel

Roles and responsibilities of EMS personnel include the following:

- Maintain the readiness of all equipment, including disinfecting, packaging, and storing.
- Monitor personal safety, patient safety, and the safety of others on the scene.
- Evaluate the scene for additional resources when indicated.
- Gain access to the patient only when it is safe to do so
- Perform an assessment of the patient's condition and needs.
- Provide emergency medical care as needed (or until additional resources arrive).
- Provide emotional support to the patient, family, and other providers.
- Maintain the continuity of care.
- Ensure that medical and legal standards are upheld and that patient privacy is protected.
- Communicate with others and maintain community relations.

- Practice professional behavior (integrity, self-motivation, self-confidence, tact, respect, and professional appearance).
- Maintain certification and meet continuing education requirements.

NATIONAL EMS EDUCATION AGENDA FOR THE FUTURE: A SYSTEMS APPROACH

The **National EMS Education Agenda for the Future: A Systems Approach** proposed an education system for EMS with five primary components, establishing the following goals for 2010 and 2020:

1. Core content: Core content to be developed by the EMS medical community, educators, and providers under leadership of the National Highway Traffic Safety Administration (NHTSA) to ensure consistency of content and reciprocity of certification. The core content should be tied to licensure and accreditation.
2. Scope-of-practice model: National models to be used by states for all levels of EMS certification/licensure.
3. Education standards: Standards that are developed by EMS educators with input from the medical community and regulators and that are peer reviewed.
4. Education program accreditation: A single national accreditation agency will develop standards and guidelines.
5. EMS certification: Four levels of national certification with different educational requirements, standards, scopes of practice, and certification: (1) entry-level emergency medical responder (EMR), (2) next-level emergency medical technician (EMT), (3) advanced AEMT (AEMT), and (4) paramedic.

QUALITY IMPROVEMENT

Quality improvement requires that an organization or system continually evaluates processes and outcomes and takes measures to improve the quality of care. The focus of quality improvement is on patient safety in access, provision of care, transport, and hand-off. Errors are often related to these different types of failures:

- Skills-based: Includes slips and mistakes. Slips occur when the AEMT has the correct intent but does not carry out an action as intended, such as mistakenly using the wrong piece of equipment. Mistakes occur when the AEMT has an incorrect intention that leads to incorrect action.
- Rules-based: The AEMT incorrectly applies a rule, applies a bad or wrong rule, or fails to apply the correct rules. For example, an AEMT is injured because of failing to assess safety before approaching a patient.
- Knowledge-based: The AEMT's knowledge is not adequate for the situation.

EMS personnel can help reduce errors by debriefing, constantly reevaluating and questioning assumptions, using established protocols and decision aids, and asking for assistance when needed.

CONTINUOUS QUALITY IMPROVEMENT (CQI)

Continuous quality improvement (CQI) emphasizes the organization and systems and processes within that organization rather than emphasizing individuals. It recognizes internal customers (staff) and external customers (patients) and uses data to improve processes. CQI represents the concept that most processes can be improved. CQI uses the scientific method of experimentation to meet needs and improve services and uses various tools, such as brainstorming, multivoting, various charts and diagrams, storyboarding, and meetings. Core concepts include the following:

- Quality and success are meeting or exceeding internal and external customers' needs and expectations.
- Problems relate to processes, and variations in processes lead to variations in results.
- Change can be made in small steps.

Steps to CQI include the following:

- Forming a knowledgeable team.
- Identifying and defining measures used to determine success.
- Brainstorming strategies for change.
- Plan, collect, and use data as part of making decisions.
- Test changes and revise or refine as needed.

RESEARCH

Research is especially important in identifying the need for changes in procedures and protocols in order to improve patient outcomes. Research depends on the gathering of data. Data collection may include direct observations, surveys, interviews, and various other sources of information, such as documents and audiovisual materials. Literature research requires a comprehensive evaluation of current (≤ 5 years) and/or historical information. Most literature research begins with an Internet search of databases, which provides listings of books, journals, and other materials on specific topics. Databases vary in content, and many contain only a reference listing with or without an abstract, so once the listing is obtained, the researcher must do a further search (publisher, library, etc.) to locate the material. Some databases require a subscription, but access is often available through educational or healthcare institutions. In order to search effectively, the researcher should begin by writing a brief explanation of the research to help identify possible keywords and synonyms to use as search words.

EVIDENCE-BASED DECISION MAKING

Although traditional medical practice has been based on knowledge, intuition, and judgment, these practices have not always been supported by evidence. **Evidence-based decision making** results in best practices based on best evidence. Steps include the following:

- Formulating a question regarding treatment and/or procedures.
- Conducting a search of the appropriate medical literature, often beginning with the search of an online database to find research that is related to the question.
- Determining the validity (measure of accuracy) and reliability (consistency) of the evidence. Evaluating the level of evidence (1a and 1b are the most valid, and 1c is required by state or federal regulations or is an industry standard).
- Assessing data (information) to determine if they apply to current needs.
- Drawing up a plan for change with input from all staff members.
- Implementing changes.
- Monitoring changes and outcomes.

METHODS OF DATA COLLECTION

When developing **data collection procedures** to determine needs, the following must be considered: the purpose of the data collection, the audience for which the data are intended, the types of questions to be answered, the scope of the research, and the resources available to carry out data collection.

Method	Issues regarding procedures
Direct observation	Observers must be selected and trained on how to observe and when and how to record observations.
Interviews	Interview questions must be developed and validated, and the interviewers must be given practice time.
Questionnaires	The type of questionnaire, the questions, and the Likert scale must be determined as well as the method of distribution (one-on-one, group, email, Internet).
Record review	A form or checklist should be developed to guide record review, and the records should be selected based on criteria established for the research.

Method	Issues regarding procedures
Secondary analysis	The databases to be mined should be selected, and the criteria for the research should be established, including keywords, time frames, and populations.

PERSONAL PROTECTIVE EQUIPMENT (PPE)

Personal protective equipment (PPE) should be readily available in the appropriate sizes for each EMS individual.

- Gowns: Should be worn for risk of splash or spray with body fluids (severe bleeding, childbirth) and should be fluid resistant.
- Eye protectors: Should be worn for risk of splash or spray with body fluids or contact with debris, such as at a worksite or in a collapsing building. Goggles should fit snugly and have antifog features. (Prescription eyeglasses do not take the place of goggles.)
- Face shields: Provide protection for face, eyes, nose, and mouth. These are preferred to goggles when there is risk of spray or splash of body fluids. They should wrap around and cover the forehead and extend to below the chin.
- Masks: Protect the nose and mouth from fluids and particles and should be fluid resistant, fit snugly, and have a flexible nosepiece.
- Respirators (such as N95, N99, and N100): Protect the nose, mouth, and airway passages exposed to hazardous or infectious aerosols, including bacteria (tuberculosis [TB], measles patients).

HAND HYGIENE AND GLOVES

Hand hygiene should be done before eating, before and after direct contact with a patient's skin, after contact with any body fluids, after contact with inanimate objects in the patient's immediate vicinity, when moving hands from a dirty to a clean area, after removing gloves, and after using the restroom.

Hand hygiene is carried out in the following two manners:

- Antiseptic soaps/detergents: For visible soiling, after exposure to diarrhea stool or a patient with diarrhea, before eating, and after using the restroom. Wet hands, apply product, rub hands together vigorously for 15 seconds, covering all surfaces, rinse hands with water, and use a disposable towel to dry them.
- Alcohol-based hand sanitizers (the most effective way to kill bacteria): For all other situations. Apply product and rub hands together, including between the fingers, for about 20 seconds until the skin surfaces are dry.

Gloves must be worn when touching any body fluids, nonintact skin, open wounds, or mucous membranes (eyes, mouth, nose); gloves should be changed when moving from a dirty area to a clean one or from one patient to another.

PROCEDURES FOR EXPOSURE/CONTAMINATION

Any **exposure/contamination** should be reported at hand-off and to the appropriate infection control person following protocols, and follow-up care should be sought if necessary. Decontamination procedures are as follows:

- Skin: Cleanse the area thoroughly with soap and water.
- Eyes: Flush with water for 20 minutes.
- Needlestick: Wash the area with soap and water and report immediately.

- <u>Clothing:</u> Remove the clothing as soon as possible, and wash visible soiling of skin with soap and water if a shower is not immediately available, but shower as soon as possible. Clothes should be washed separately in a washing machine at the workplace.
- <u>Equipment/Vehicle:</u> Clean thoroughly with disinfectant. Dispose of equipment if unable to adequately decontaminate it.

When reporting exposures/contamination, note the type of exposure, the date and time of exposure, circumstances, actions taken to decontaminate, and any other required information.

ISOLATION GUIDELINES

The **2007 CDC Guideline for Isolation Precautions** includes the standard precautions that apply to all patients and transmission-based precautions for those with known or suspected infections. **Standard precautions** should be used for all patients because all body fluids (sweat, urine, feces, blood, and sputum) and nonintact skin and mucous membranes may be infected.

Hand hygiene	Wash hands before and after each patient contact and after any contact with body fluids and contaminated items. Use soap and water for visible soiling.
Protective equipment	Use personal protective equipment (PPE), such as gloves, gowns, and masks, eye protection, and/or face shields, when anticipating contact with body fluids or contaminated skin.
Respiratory hygiene/ Cough etiquette	Use source-control measures, such as covering cough, disposing of tissues, using a surgical mask on the person coughing or on staff to prevent inhalation of droplets, and properly disposing of dressings and used equipment. Wash hands after contacting respiratory secretions. Maintain a distance of >3 feet from a coughing person when possible.
Sharps	Dispose of sharps, such as needles, carefully in sharps containers. Do not recap needles.

TRANSMISSION-BASED PRECAUTIONS

The **2007 CDC Guideline for Isolation Precautions** includes the standard precautions that apply to all patients and **transmission-based precautions** for those with known or suspected infections as well as those with excessive wound drainage, other discharge, or fecal incontinence. Transmission-based precautions include the following:

Contact	Use PPE, including gown and gloves, for all contacts with the patient or the patient's immediate environment.
Droplet	(Appropriate for influenza, streptococcus infection, pertussis, rhinovirus, and adenovirus and pathogens that remain viable and infectious for only short distances.) Use a mask while caring for the patient. Maintain the patient at a distance of >3 feet away from other patients (with a curtain separating them in an emergency department). Use a patient mask if transporting a patient.
Airborne	(Appropriate for measles, chickenpox, tuberculosis, and severe acute respiratory syndrome [SARS] because pathogens remain viable and infectious for long distances.) Use ≥N95 respirators (or masks) while caring for the patient. The patient should be placed in an airborne infection isolation room in an emergency department.

IMMUNIZATIONS FOR EMS PERSONNEL

The Centers for Disease Control and Prevention (CDC) recommends the following **immunizations** for all healthcare workers, including EMS personnel:

- Hepatitis B: Three-dose series (now, in one month, and five months later) followed by an anti-HBs serologic test 30 to 60 days after the third immunization.
- Measles, mumps, rubella (MMR): Two-dose series with the second immunization at least 28 days after the first for those born during or after 1957 and those born before 1957 without proof of immunity.
- Varicella (chickenpox): Two doses, four weeks apart. (A combined MMRV immunization is available.)
- Influenza: Annually.
- Tetanus, diphtheria, and pertussis (Tdap): One time with a tetanus (TD) booster every 10 years. The TD injection does not protect against pertussis (whooping cough).
- Meningococcal: One dose.

Screening for tuberculosis with a chest x-ray or skin test is also recommended.

STRESS

The AEMT must often deal with **stressful incidents**, such as dangerous situations (storm conditions, gunshots, falling debris); critically ill patients; unpleasant sights, sounds, and odors; multipatient incidents; and angry/upset patients, family members, and bystanders. The AEMT should not argue or become defensive but should remain calm and supportive, allowing the patient to express his or her feelings and trying to defuse the situation while administering medical care and cooperating with other first responders. If a patient has no pulse or respirations and does not have a valid do-not-resuscitate (DNR) order, the AEMT should attempt resuscitation unless doing so puts the AEMT at risk; the injuries are not compatible with life; or obvious signs of death are present, such as tissue decay, livor mortis, which is discoloration in the lowermost blood vessels from pooled blood shortly after death, or rigor mortis, which is stiffening of the joints that occurs within 2 to 6 hours of death (verified by checking two or more joints). After 24 to 48 hours of rigor mortis, the muscles become flaccid.

Warning signs of stress often begin with difficulty sleeping and nightmares about work, loss of appetite, and lack of interest in usual activities, including work and intimacy. The individual may feel increasingly sad and depressed and may have difficulty concentrating, making decisions, and carrying out tasks. The individual may also begin to isolate from others and exhibit irritability with coworkers, family, and friends. Some individuals develop physical symptoms related to stress, such as stomach upset, headaches, nausea, and high blood pressure (BP), whereas others may experience panic attacks. Some individuals may try to self-medicate with alcohol or drugs. When experiencing the warning signs of stress, the individual should talk about the problems with someone trusted, such as a physician, coworker, supervisor, or family member, and he or she may need to seek assistance from a professional counselor. Lifestyle changes, such as decreasing the use of alcohol or drugs, exercising regularly, and practicing relaxation exercises, may help to relieve stress.

Stress reactions include the following:

- Acute stress reaction: This reaction usually occurs quickly (minutes to hours) in response to an event that is stressful (such as the death of a child or a multiple-casualty incident). The individual may experience physical symptoms (with the release of adrenaline) such as rapid pulse, nausea, chest tightness, headache, fast respirations, and increased perspiration. An acute stress reaction usually recedes quickly, but it may persist for weeks in some individuals.
- Delayed stress reaction: Although the individual may cope well with a stressful event initially, months later, the person may begin to have nightmares, anxiety, and other indications of post-traumatic stress.

- Cumulative stress reaction: This type of stress reaction occurs when the individual has repeated stressors (either in the workplace or in his or her personal life) that cause repeated acute stress reactions, resulting in various physical and psychological problems. This is especially common in EMS personnel.

PREVENTION OF RESPONSE-RELATED INJURIES
Prevention of response-related injuries includes the following:

- Infectious diseases: Use PPE and understand the spread of infectious diseases—air (coughing), direct contact (blood, vomitus, other body fluids), needlestick, contaminated food/equipment, and sexual transmission. Maintain current immunizations.
- Personal habits: Obtain adequate sleep, nutrition, and exercise. Avoid excessive alcohol and tobacco.
- Environmental hazards: Conduct a 360° assessment. Note traffic hazards, the vehicle's condition, fire, leaking fluids, downed power lines, hazardous materials (look for placards and warning symbols; avoid the area until it is cleared). Use PPE and respirators as indicated.
- Violence: Defuse situations, make a safe response (assistance of law enforcement), and use restraints if necessary for dangerous or violent individuals.
- Collisions: Drive safely; avoid speeding and driving through stop signs and red lights when possible. Wear seat belts and/or safety harnesses.

END OF LIFE/DEATH AND DYING
Grief is a normal response to the death or severe illness/abnormality of a patient. How a person deals with grief is very personal, and each will grieve differently. Elisabeth Kübler-Ross identified **five stages of grief**, which can apply to patients and family members. A person may not go through each stage, but he or she usually goes through two of the five stages.

Stage	Patient/Family	Appropriate AEMT response
1. Denial	Resistive to information, stunned, immobile, detached, unable to respond appropriately	Be patient and supportive and repeat information as needed.
2. Anger	Lashing out, overt hostility, self-blame, blaming others	Do not respond in anger or take statements personally; remain calm and supportive, but be alert to the risk of physical attack.
3. Bargaining	If–then thinking, demanding another opinion or expert, praying	Avoid making any judgmental statements.
4. Depression	Tearful, crying, withdrawn, sad, isolated	Encourage expression of feelings, remain supportive, and assure the individual that these feelings are normal.
5. Acceptance	Resolution	Listen patiently and remain supportive.

SIGNS AND SYMBOLS

Sign/Symbol	Interpretation
	Flame: Includes flammable materials and gases and those that are self-heating or self-reactive.
	Corrosion: Includes substances that can cause skin burns, metal corrosion, and eye damage.
	Health hazard: Includes carcinogens, toxic substances, and respiratory irritants.
	Poison: Includes materials, gases, or substances that are extremely toxic and may result in death or severe illness.
	Irritant: Includes material, gases, or substances that are irritants to skin, eyes, and/or respiratory tract, are acutely toxic, or have a narcotic effect.
	Biohazard: Includes biological substances, such as body fluids, that pose a threat to humans. Appears on sharps containers that hold contaminated needles.

PRINCIPLES OF BODY MECHANICS

Basic principles of body mechanics include the following:

- Avoid reaching for prolonged periods of time, overhead, or more than 20 inches away.
- Avoid pulling—push, roll, or slide instead.
- Avoid lifting—push, roll, or slide instead.
- Lift with leg muscles, not with the back.
- Hold weight close to the body rather than at arm's length.
- Flex at the hips and knees, not the waist.
- Carry patients head first upstairs and feet first downstairs.
- Maintain a straight back and avoid twisting.
- Assess weight and recognize limitations in lifting/carrying.
- Get help when necessary, and communicate every step with your partner ("Lift on the count of three").
- Maintain a firm base of support with feet apart (shoulder width) to stabilize your stance.

- Maintain the line of gravity (the imaginary line between your center of gravity and the ground) within the base of support.
- Position yourself close to an object that is to be lifted or carried.
- Lift patients from stable ground.

MOVING AND LIFTING PATIENTS

Techniques for moving patients include the following:

- Direct ground lift: Use only for lightweight individuals with no suspected spinal injuries. Three rescuers line up on one side of the patient, and each kneels on the same knee. The AEMT at the head places one arm under the patient's neck and shoulder and the other arm under the patient's lower back. The middle AEMT places his or her arms above and below the patient's waist, and the AEMT at the patient's feet places his or her arms under the knees and lower legs. On the count of three, they roll the patient onto their knees and toward their chests. On the count of three, they stand and move the patient.
- Power lift: Place feet (shoulder width) apart and pointing slightly outward; tighten the back and abdominal muscles. Squat down as though sitting. Place hands 10 inches apart with the palms upward (power grip) while grasping the stretcher and lift with the upper body becoming vertical before the hips rise.
- Extremity lift: Requires two AEMTs. One AEMT squats at the patient's head and another is at one side by the patient's knees. The AEMT at the head folds the patient's arms across the chest and grasps the patient by wrapping both arms around the torso under the patient's arms and grasping the patient's wrists. The second AEMT slides his or her hands beneath the patient's knees and lower legs, and together they stand and lift the patient.
- Squat lift: Requires two AEMTs. One AEMT squats with the back straight and the weak foot slightly forward at the head of patient, and the other AEMT is in the same position at the patient's feet. Grasp the patient's upper body as for the extremity lift and grasp the patient's feet. Both AEMTs push up with the stronger foot and lift with the upper body becoming vertical before the hips rise.
- Logroll: Used to position carrying devices under the patient and for some transfers; it requires two AEMTs positioned on the same side of the patient. Place the patient's arm on the side that he or she is being turned to above his or her head or over the chest. Place the patient's other arm across his or her chest. If on the ground, squat close to the patient. The AEMT at the patient's head reaches across the patient and grasps his or her shoulders and trunk while the second AEMT grasps his or her trunk and legs. On the count of three, they turn the patient in one smooth move.
- Draw-sheet transfer: Requires four AEMTs with two positioned on one side of the patient and two positioned on the other side but on the opposite side of the bed or stretcher to which the patient will be transferred. The logroll technique is used to place a draw sheet under the patient. AEMTs on both sides roll the edges of the draw sheet until the edges are close to the patient. On the count of three, they lift the patient slightly and move the patient across to the bed.

BACKBOARDS AND CERVICAL COLLARS

Backboards were originally designed to transfer patients. However, **backboards and cervical collars** have been routinely used for EMS rescues for many years without evidence-based studies supporting their use. The premise was that stabilizing the spine and neck would prevent further injury in case a spinal injury had occurred, but spinal injuries are relatively rare, and some studies indicate that these devices do not provide any protection and, in fact, may cause damage. Additionally, cervical collars restrict the airway by 20% or more and may worsen injuries if not properly sized for the patient. Because of these findings, some EMS no longer routinely use backboards but use a vacuum mattress in a scoop basket instead. The American Association of Neurological Surgeons/Congress of Neurological Surgeons (AANS/CNS) guidelines advise that spinal immobilization using a backboard be reserved for known or suspected spinal cord injury without penetrating injury, although the use of the cervical collar is still recommended until the cervical spine is assessed for injury. Short backboards may be used to support a patient's back in a sitting position.

RESTRAINTS

Restraints should be avoided if possible, although if a combative patient poses a risk to him- or herself or EMS personnel, restraints may be necessary to safely assess, treat, and transport the patient, keeping in mind that the altered state of consciousness may result from drug or alcohol use; traumatic injury; or from a mental or physical disorder, such as schizophrenia, dementia, or hypoglycemia (insulin reaction). Protocols for use of restraints must be followed, and restraints should be applied under medical direction. If possible, the police should be present and there should be one EMS personnel for each limb, staying beyond the limb's range of motion until ready to secure the limb, with one AEMT talking to the patient and explaining the procedure. The AEMT should avoid unnecessary force, which may result in increased combativeness and injury to the patient or others. Patients should not be restrained in the prone (face-down) position. Documentation must include the reason for restraining the patient, the time, and the method of restraint.

Common **types of physical restraints** include the following:

- Soft: Padded cuffs (often leather) that fasten about the wrists and ankles and are attached to a long board. These are the most commonly used restraints.
- Stretcher/Spinal board straps: These may be strapped across the chest (not too tight), abdomen, or legs to help restrict movement.
- Long board/Spinal board: Patient should be restrained to the long board and then placed on a wheeled stretcher and never tied to or fastened to the stretcher.
- Spit sock: A hood that fits over the patient's head to prevent him or her from biting or spitting.
- Cervical collar: This is used to protect the patient's cervical spine and to prevent him or her from biting.

The AEMT should not place the patient in handcuffs or hard plastic ties. If these were placed on a patient by a law enforcement officer and must stay in place, such as with a criminal or an extremely violent patient, then a law enforcement officer must stay with the patient at all times.

EMERGENCY MOVES

Emergency moves may be needed if the patient and/or AEMT is in immediate danger from fire, explosives, or other hazards; if the patient requires life-saving treatment, such as cardiopulmonary resuscitation (CPR); or if the patient is in water, such as a pond or lake. Emergency moves include the following:

- Blanket drag: Logroll the patient onto a blanket, wrap the patient in the blanket, grasp the blanket near the patient's head while in a squatting position with your back straight, and drag. If there are two rescuers, the other should be positioned at the patient's feet and should be pushing.
- Clothing drag: Squat down by the patient's head, securely grasp the clothing near the patient's neck or shoulders (avoid grasping by a T-shirt), and drag the patient.
- Arm drag: Squat down by the patient's head. Fold the patient's arms across his or her chest. Grasp the patient under the arms, wrapping your arms about the torso and grasping the patient's wrists to stabilize his or her arms. Drag the patient.

Urgent moves, such as with altered mental status, shock, or breathing difficulties, should also be done as quickly as possible.

Emergency moves can be carried out by one rescuer if no other assistance is available, as follows:

- Firefighter's drag: Tie the patient's wrists together with any available material. Straddle the patient and pull the patient's arms over your neck and then crawl forward, dragging him or her beneath you.

- Firefighter's carry: Grasp the patient's knees and pull them together and up. Stand on the patient's feet and reach out and grab one of the patient's arms with one hand. Pull the patient upright, and, as the patient elevates, place your other hand between the patient's legs. Place the patient's arm behind your neck and continue to pull the patient and lift until he or she is draped across your upper back with the arm hanging free. Then grasp the patient's arm that is hanging with the hand that is between the legs to secure the patient.

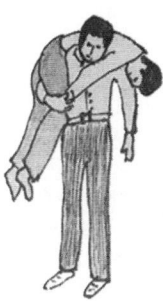

Minimum Data Sets

Minimum data sets are the minimum data specifically required for EMS services. These consist of the following:

- Patient information: This derives from the assessment including the patient's primary complaint and the findings during the initial assessment—the patient's name and address; vital signs (blood pressure [BP], pulse [P], and respiration rate [R]); and descriptions of any wounds, injuries, pain, or other symptoms. The patient's demographics (age, gender, ethnic background) should be noted as well as any other identifying or essential information.
- Administrative information: This includes the time of the initial report, time the EMS unit was notified, time of arrival at the incident, time of leaving the scene, time of arrival at the destination (hospital, trauma center), and time of hand-off.
- Accurate/Synchronous clocks: All members of the EMS system should use accurate and synchronous clocks so that they all are set to the same time to ensure there is no disparity in time reporting.

Prehospital Care Report

The **prehospital care report** serves as a legal document to show that emergent care was provided. It describes the condition of the patient upon the AEMT's arrival at the scene, interventions provided, and changes in the patient's condition; it is essential to ensure continuity of care. The documenting AEMT may be called in to legal proceedings. The prehospital care report may also be used for educational purposes, such as through debriefing and case review. Additionally, the report is used administratively as the basis for billing as well as for the collection of data for research and evaluation of continuous quality improvement. Required elements of documentation include the time of events (receipt of call, arrival at incident, time of transport, arrival at destination), assessment findings (vital signs, injuries, bleeding, mental status), emergent care, changes in the patient's condition, response to the treatment provided, scene observations (specific place/area), hazards, and disposition of patient (care refusal, transportation, hand-off). Documentation may be on paper or may be done electronically and may combine checkboxes and narrative reports. Run data are those data elements that are required for reporting of each run.

Narrative Documentation

With **narrative documentation**, the AEMT should take care not to repeat the same information already provided in checkboxes. The AEMT should describe what was observed directly rather than the conclusions based on those observations and should record all pertinent information and observations, avoiding nonstandardized abbreviations and radio codes, which may be misunderstood or misinterpreted. Any pertinent negatives, such as patient or family complaints, must be documented. If the incident has legal implications, such as in the case of assault, any pertinent comments or sensitive information ("I was raped") should be quoted directly and the source should be noted. Care should be taken to write clearly and spell correctly. Time should be documented for every intervention and reassessment. Any state or local reporting requirements must be met in documentation, and the contents of the prehospital report should remain confidential and be distributed only to appropriate healthcare providers. No data may be falsified, and any errors and steps taken to correct those errors must be documented.

Patient Refusal of Medical Care

According to the **Patient Self-Determination Act** (1990), competent patients have the right to refuse any medical treatment, and parents have the right to make this decision for minor children. If a patient refuses care, then the AEMT should try to persuade the patient to go to the hospital by giving the reasons and possible consequences of refusal. The patient should be asked to sign the refusal form, and a family member, police officer, or bystander should sign as a witness to the patient's signing or witness the patient's refusal to sign. The AEMT should complete documentation of any assessment carried out and any refusal of the patient to assessment. The AEMT should carefully document the conversation between the AEMT and patient regarding refusal of care and consequences and should document the proposed care as well as the information the AEMT gave the patient about alternate care (such as a visit to the personal physician) and the willingness to return if the patient has a change of mind.

Special Situations

Documentation errors: In handwritten documents, draw one line through the error, initial, and write the correct information beside the error. If information was omitted, add a note with the date and your initials. If documentation was electronic, follow the method prescribed for corrections.

Multiple-casualty incidents: Record information temporarily for later complete documentation, if necessary, following the procedures in place for such an incident.

Incident reports: Fill out forms as soon as possible, document any witnesses to the incident, and file forms according to protocol. Incident reports are often maintained separately from prehospital reports.

Special-situation reports: Used for events/incidents that must be reported to an outside authority or as a supplement to the prehospital report. Fill out the report as soon as possible, and include the names of all parties involved; use objective descriptions, and avoid stating conclusions. Maintain a personal copy.

Transfer reports: Ensure that they contain minimum data sets and provide a transfer signature. These are used during hand-off.

EMS System Communication

With the **AEMT's arrival** at the scene of an incident, he or she should assess the situation and the need for added resources, such as additional EMS personnel or police, and contact the appropriate authorities to request assistance. When additional EMS personnel arrive or contact is made with medical control or the receiving facility, the AEMT should self-identify and provide a verbal report of the patient's current condition, including demographic information such as age and gender. The AEMT should report the patient's chief complaint and provide any history that is pertinent as well as the condition of the patient on arrival and any history of major illnesses. The AEMT should also report the results of the patient assessment, including the vital signs and any physical/psychological findings, as well as any treatment provided and the patient's response to the treatment. The AEMT should communicate with law enforcement officers and other responders, such as firefighters, especially regarding safety concerns.

Components of an EMS communication system include the base station of a two-way radio system, which is in a fixed location, such as a dispatch center. The base station facilitates communication among a number of hand-held/mobile radios. There is often only one channel per base station, so additional base stations may be installed to add more channels. Radio transmitters/receivers may be vehicular mounted or mobile, although mobile transmitters/receivers may have limited range because they tend to have lower power (1–5 watts) than do base stations (20–50 watts). Typically, the mobile device has a range of 10– preserve evidence15 miles over average terrain, but it is shorter in rugged terrain. The Federal Communications Commission (FCC) controls radio frequencies, and those used for EMS are in the public safety pool.

COMMUNICATION WITH MEDICAL CONTROL

The AEMT may be in **communication with medical control** regarding a patient's condition and need for medication. Medical control may be at the receiving facility or at a separate site. Upon receiving an order by phone or radio, the AEMT should repeat back the order and dosage to ensure that the message was received correctly. When using the radio, the radio must be turned on and the press-to-talk (PTT) button must be pressed before beginning transmission. The AEMT should address the medical control person by name and give the name of the AEMT's unit. Transmissions should be brief and to the point, avoiding unnecessary pleasantries, codes, agency-specific terms, profanity, and meaningless phrases, keeping in mind that the airways are public. The AEMT should give individual digits for long numbers, use "affirmative" and "negative" in place of "yes" and "no," and say "over" when the transmission is finished. Reports should be objective rather than opinion based and should avoid offering a diagnosis. The dispatcher must be notified when the unit leaves the scene.

PHONE/CELLULAR COMMUNICATION AND INTERPERSONAL COMMUNICATION WITH PATIENTS

Phone/Cellular communication: This is similar to radio communication, but the

AEMT should be familiar with important phone numbers (such as medical control, hospitals, trauma centers) or have the numbers prominently posted for access. The AEMT should also be aware of dead spots that may prevent communication and should have a backup plan (radio) for when cellular transmission fails.

Interpersonal communication: Upon arrival at the scene of an incident, the AEMT should self-introduce, making eye contact, and he or she should communicate using language that the patient can understand, that is age-appropriate, and that avoids any medical jargon. The AEMT should be positioned at or below the level of the patient if possible to avoid intimidating the patient and should remain aware of body language. The AEMT should be honest and speak slowly and calmly, using the patient's first or last name, depending on the age of the patient and the circumstances. The AEMT may request interpreters if necessary.

EFFECTIVE COMMUNICATION AND INTERVIEWING TECHNIQUES

Effective communication begins with a self-introduction and an introduction of other team members to the patient and family and includes respecting the patient's privacy by shielding the patient from passersby if possible and avoiding loudly repeating any patient information. If possible, the AEMT should adjust lighting and limit outside distractions such as noise. When interviewing the patient, the AEMT should ask open-ended questions (such as "Can you describe your pain?") and avoid questions that can be answered with "yes" or "no." The AEMT should ask direct questions, such as "When did the pain start?" Questions should be asked one at a time while allowing the patient/family time to respond. It's especially important to observe the patient's body language (posture, eye contact, gestures, and tone of voice) to determine if it matches his or her words and to avoid medical/professional jargon. The AEMT should avoid giving false reassurances or advice and should avoid leading/biased questions, being too talkative, interrupting the patient, and asking "why" questions, such as "Why did you take an overdose of medication?"

SPECIAL INTERVIEW SITUATIONS

Interviewing **hostile patients** requires a calm response, avoiding negative responses and using reflective statements, such as "I can understand your feelings." The AEMT should maintain eye contact (50% to 60% of the time) and try to defuse the situation, but he or she should avoid staring or standing too close and having crossed arms because this may be misinterpreted as threatening behavior. If patients are **sexually aggressive**, it's important to tell them that the behavior is inappropriate and to ask them to stop. When interviewing patients under the **influence of drugs or alcohol,** try to ask essential questions such as the type and amount of drug/alcohol ingested. Obtain information from family or friends if necessary. When patients are **hearing impaired**, the AEMT should face the person directly, speak slowly and distinctly (but avoid shouting), provide information in writing if possible, use pantomime, and try to reduce environmental noise. Knowledge of the alphabet in sign language can be very useful to communicate with the deaf, especially if a sign-language translator is unavailable.

When **interviewing elderly patients**, the AEMT should be alert to possible cognitive, hearing, or vision impairments, especially if the patient appears confused upon questioning or his or her answers are inappropriate. The AEMT should ask if the patient has eyeglasses or a hearing aid and should obtain them if possible. The patient's family may be able to assist with the interview. If the patient's speech is unclear, he or she may need to put in dentures. When communicating with a **pediatric patient**, the AEMT should have the parent or caregiver comfort the child and answer questions, especially if the child is an infant or is very young. The AEMT should use simple sentences and age-appropriate language and explain to the child what he or she is doing to help alleviate the child's fear. Adolescents should be addressed directly even if a parent or caregiver is providing some information, and, in some cases, the adolescent will provide more information if the parent/caregiver is not present.

DYNAMICS OF THE COMMUNICATION PROCESS

The **communication process**, which includes the sender-receiver feedback loop, is based on Claude Shannon's article, "A Mathematical Theory of Communication" (1948), in which he provided the basis for information theory and described three necessary steps of successful communication: encoding a message, transmitting it through a channel, and decoding it. The resultant communication process begins with the sender, who serves as the encoder and determines the content of the message. The medium is the form the message takes (digital, written, audiovisual), and the channel is the method of delivery (mail, radio, TV, phone, email, text message). The recipient (receiver), who acts as the decoder, determines the meaning from the message. Feedback helps to determine whether or not the communication is successful and whether the message is understood as intended. This process is referred to as the sender-receiver feedback loop. Context is the environment (physical and psychological) in which the communication occurs, and interference is any factor that impacts the communication process. Interference may be external (such as environmental noise) or internal (such as emotional distress or anxiety).

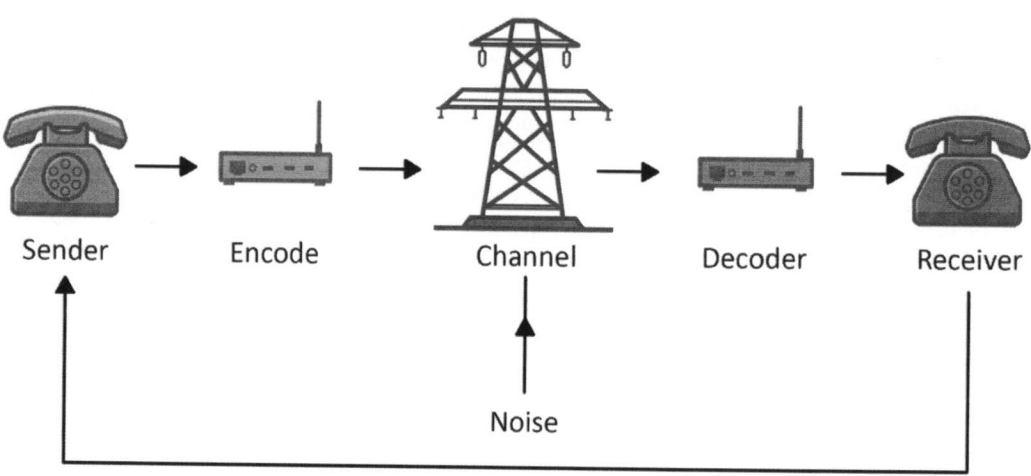

Therapeutic Communication

Therapeutic communication begins with respect for the individual/family and the assumption that all communication, verbal and nonverbal, has meaning. Listening must be done empathetically. Techniques that facilitate communication include the following:

Introduction	Make a personal introduction and use the individual's name: "Mrs. Brown, I am Toby Williams, your AEMT."
Encouragement	Use an open-ended opening question: "Is there anything you'd like to discuss?" Acknowledge comments: Say "yes" and "I understand." Allow silence and observe nonverbal behavior rather than trying to force a conversation. Ask for clarification if the patient's statements are unclear. Reflect the patient's statements back (use sparingly): Individual: "I hate this hospital." AEMT: "You hate this hospital?"
Empathy	Make observations: "You are shaking," and "You seem worried." Recognize feelings: Individual: "I want to get well." AEMT: "It must be hard for you to deal with this illness." Provide information as honestly and completely as possible about the patient's condition, treatment, and procedures and respond to the individual's questions and concerns.
Exploration	Verbally express implied messages: Individual: "This treatment is too much trouble." AEMT: "Do you think the treatment isn't helping you?" Explore a topic, but allow the individual to terminate the discussion without further probing: "I'd like to hear how you feel about that."
Orientation	Indicate reality: Individual: "Someone is screaming." AEMT: "That sound was a police siren." Comment on distortions without directly agreeing or disagreeing: Individual: "That policeman promised I could go to St. John's Hospital." AEMT: "Really? That's surprising because this ambulance is based at County Hospital."
Collaboration	Work together to achieve better results: "Maybe if we talk about this, we can figure out a way to make the treatment easier for you."
Validation	Seek validation: "Do you feel better now?" or "Did the medication help you breathe better?"

Cultural Considerations

Hmong	The eldest male in the family makes the decisions for the family and is deferred to by other family members, so the AEMT should ask who should receive information about the patient. Communication should be polite and respectful, avoiding direct eye contact, which is considered rude. Disagreeing is considered rude, so "yes" may mean "I hear you" and NOT "I agree with you."
Mexican	Mexican culture perceives time with more flexibility than does American culture, so if patients/family need to be present at a particular time, the AEMT should specify the exact time ("be here at 1:30 PM") and explain the reason rather than saying something that is more vague, such as "be here after lunch." People may appear to be unassertive or unable to make decisions when they are simply showing respect to the AEMT by being deferent. In traditional families, the males make decisions, so a woman may wait for the husband or other males in the family to make decisions about her treatment or care.

Middle Eastern	In Middle Eastern countries, males make the decisions, so issues for discussion or decision should be directed to males, such as the patient's spouse or son, and males may be direct in stating what they want, sometimes appearing demanding. Middle Easterners often require less personal space and may stand very close. If a male AEMT must care for a female patient, then the family should be advised that *only* medical treatments, not personal care, will be done by the male AEMT.
Asian	Asian families may expect the AEMT to remain authoritative and to give directions and may not question the AEMT's authority. Disagreeing is considered impolite. "Yes" may only mean that the person is heard, not that they agree with the person. When asked if they understand, they may indicate that they do even when they clearly do not so as not to offend the AEMT. Asians may avoid eye contact as an indication of respect.

CULTURAL COMPETENCE

There are a number of issues related to cultural competence in communicating with others.

- **Eye contact:** Many cultures use eye contact differently than what is common in the United States. Some patients and families, such as Asians, Native Americans, and Arabs, may avoid direct eye contact, considering it rude, or they may look away to signal disapproval or may look down to signal respect. Careful observation of the way family members use eye contact can help to determine what will be most comfortable for the patient/family.
- **Distance**: Some cultures stand close to others (<4 feet) when speaking (Middle Easterners, Hispanics), and others stand at a greater distance (>4 feet) (Northern Europeans, many Americans). There is a considerable difference relating to concepts of personal space among cultures. Allowing the family to approach or observing whether they tend to move closer, lean forward, or move back can help to determine a comfortable distance for communication.
- **Time**: Americans tend to be time oriented, and they expect people to be on time, but time is viewed more flexibly in many other cultures.

INTERVIEWING TECHNIQUES

If possible, the patient should be interviewed alone or should be asked if he or she wants family members present. Verbal and nonverbal responses should be observed during **an interview.** Information should include not only the patient's facts but also the patient's attitude and concerns. The AEMT should ask one question at a time in language that the patient understands and avoid providing false reassurances and advice or interrupting. Strategies include the following:

- Ask open-ended informational questions (as opposed to yes/no) with "who," "what," "where," "when," and "how," but avoid questions with "why" if possible.
    - Instead of "Why do you continue to use heroin?" ask "Have you tried to quit drug use?"
- Ask brief clarifying questions: "How long have you had weakness in your left side?"
- Provide a list of options: "Is your headache throbbing, stabbing, or dull?"
- Rephrase/reflect to encourage clarification.
    - Patient: "My husband had the same type of fall and died a month later."
    - AEMT: "You're afraid you might die from this fall."

CONDITIONS FOR CONSENT

The **conditions for consent** for care and decision-making capacity include the following:

- 18 years or older: Patients who are younger may have the right to give consent for all or some medical treatment in some states. State laws vary; for example, the age of consent for medical treatment in Alabama is 14.

- Mentally competent to make decisions: May be impaired by mental disability, injury, illness, or substance abuse (intoxication).
- Court-emancipated minor.
- Military service.
- Marriage.

Consent may be expressed if the patient is able to give informed consent, or it may be implied, such as when care is provided in an emergent situation in which the patient is unable to give consent. Parents or caregivers give consent for minors younger than the age of 18 unless they have been emancipated. If parents or caregivers are unavailable to give consent, life-saving emergent care, general medical assessment, and medical care to prevent further injury or harm can be provided without consent.

INFORMED CONSENT

Patients or their families must provide **informed consent** for all treatments that they receive. This includes a thorough explanation of all procedures and treatment and the associated risks. Patients/families should be apprised of all options and allowed input on the type of treatments. Patients/families should be apprised of all reasonable risks and any complications that might be life threatening or increase morbidity. The American Medical Association has established guidelines for informed consent as follows:

- Explanation of the diagnosis.
- Nature of and reason for the treatment or procedure.
- Risks and benefits.
- Alternative options (regardless of cost or insurance coverage).
- Risks and benefits of alternative options.
- Risks and benefits of not having a treatment or procedure.
- Providing informed consent is a requirement of all states.

The requirement for informed consent may be waived in life-threatening situations and if the AEMT cannot obtain informed consent because the patient cannot communicate and legal consent cannot be obtained.

HEALTH INSURANCE PORTABILITY AND ACCOUNTABILITY ACT OF 1996 (HIPAA)

Sensitive information is classified under the **Health Insurance Portability and Accountability Act of 1996 (HIPAA)** as protected health information (PHI), and it includes the following:

- Any information about an individual's past, present, or future health or condition (mental or physical).
- Provision of health care.
- Any identifying information related to payment for healthcare services.
- Identifying information: Name, address, Social Security number, birth date, and any document or material that contains the identifying information.

Personal information can be shared with a spouse, legal guardians, those with durable power of attorney for the patient, and those involved in the care of the patient, such as physicians, without a specific release. HIPAA mandates the following privacy and security rules to ensure that health information and individual privacy are protected:

- Privacy rule: Protected information includes any information included in the medical record (electronic or paper), conversations between the doctor and other healthcare providers, billing information, and any other form of health information.
- Security rule: Any electronic health information must be secure and protected against threats, hazards, or nonpermitted disclosure.

Advance Directives, Durable Power of Attorney, and Do-Not-Resuscitate (DNR) Order

In accordance with federal and state laws, individuals have the right to self-determination in health care, including decisions about end-of-life care through **advance directives** such as living wills and the right to assign a surrogate person to make decisions through a **durable power of attorney**. Patients should routinely be questioned about an advanced directive because they may present at a healthcare organization without the document. Patients who have indicated that they desire a **do-not-resuscitate (DNR) order** should not receive resuscitative treatments for terminal illness or conditions in which meaningful recovery cannot occur. Patients and families of those with terminal illnesses should be questioned as to whether the patients are hospice patients. For those with DNR requests or those withdrawing life support, staff should provide the patient palliative rather than curative measures, such as pain control and/or oxygen, and emotional support to the patient and family. Religious traditions and beliefs about death should be treated with respect.

Patient Refusal of Medical Care

According to the **Patient Self-Determination Act** (1990), competent patients have the right to **refusal of care,** and parents have the right to make this decision for minor children. If a patient refuses care, then the AEMT should try to persuade the patient to go to the hospital by giving the reasons and possible consequences of refusal. The patient should be asked to sign the refusal form, and a family member, police officer, or bystander should sign as a witness to the patient's signing or witness the refusal to sign. The AEMT should complete documentation of any assessment carried out and any refusal of the patient to assessment. The AEMT should carefully document the conversation between the AEMT and patient regarding refusal of care and consequences and should document the proposed care as well as the information the AEMT gave the patient about alternate care (such as a visit to the personal physician) and the willingness to return if the patient has a change of mind.

Negligence

Negligence indicates that *proper care* has not been provided, based on established standards. *Reasonable care* uses a rationale for decision-making in relation to providing care. State regulations regarding negligence may vary, but they all have some statutes of limitation, governmental immunity, and Good Samaritan laws that may provide a defense. Types of negligence include the following:

- Negligent conduct: Failure to provide reasonable care or to protect/assist another, based on existing standards and expertise.
- Gross negligence: Willfully providing inadequate care while disregarding safety/security.
- Contributory negligence: The injured party contributes to his/her own harm.
- Comparative negligence: The amount of negligence attributed to each individual involved.

If the charge of negligence is supported, the patient may collect physical (lost earnings due to injury), psychological (pain and suffering), and punitive damages.

Civil and Criminal Offenses

The four necessary elements of **negligence** (failure to follow the standards of care) are as follows:

1. Duty of care: The defendant (healthcare provider) had a duty to provide adequate care and/or protect the plaintiff's (patient's) safety.
2. Breach of duty: The defendant failed to carry out the duty to care, resulting in danger, injury, or harm to the plaintiff.
3. Damages: The plaintiff experienced illness or injury as a result of the breach of duty.
4. Causation: The plaintiff's illness or injury is directly caused by the defendant's negligent breach of duty.

Abandonment occurs if the AEMT withdraws from providing care contrary to a patient's desire or knowledge and fails to arrange for appropriate care by others, resulting in harm to the patient. **Assault** occurs if an AEMT threatens a patient in such a way that the patient becomes fearful of harm, whereas **battery** occurs when the AEMT intentionally injures a patient, such as by hitting or shoving the person. Assault and battery often occur together.

STATUTORY RESPONSIBILITIES AND MANDATORY REPORTING

The AEMT must practice within the **scope of responsibility**, which is outlined by each state's medical practice act. The AEMT must be certified/licensed according to state requirements and meet appropriate educational standards regarding preparation and continuing education. The AEMT has a duty to the patients, the medical director, and the public and functions under government and medical oversight.

Although laws about **mandatory reporting** vary from state to state, healthcare providers, including EMS personnel, are considered mandatory reporters in all states and must report suspected cases of child and elder abuse and neglect. The AEMT must follow state guidelines for reporting because simply notifying the receiving facility of suspected abuse or neglect is not adequate. The AEMT should be familiar with the signs of abuse and neglect (certain types of fractures; unexplained or multiple bruises; suspicious bruise patterns; burns; hair loss; and inadequate food, clothing, and shelter).

EVIDENCE PRESERVATION

When an incident may involve **court cases**, such as with gunshot wounds, knife, wounds, and rape, the AEMT should take steps to **preserve evidence**, although providing emergent medical care takes priority. The AEMT should try to avoid disturbing items at the scene of the incident and should assess the environment and document any unusual findings, remembering that the environment and the patient are both considered to be part of the crime scene. The AEMT should collaborate with law enforcement officers at the scene. If the patient has had a gunshot wound or a knife wound, the AEMT should not cut through the holes in the clothing but should cut along seams or away from the injuries. Any clothing or belongings removed during treatment should be secured separately in a paper bag (or plastic if paper is not available) and delivered with the patient to the receiving facility or to law enforcement officers. When the patient is describing the event, the AEMT should document using quotations rather than summarizing.

ETHICAL PRINCIPLES AND MORAL OBLIGATIONS

Ethics is a branch of philosophy that studies morality—concepts of right and wrong. Applied ethics is the use of ethical principles, such as autonomy (right to self-determination), beneficence (acting to benefit another), nonmaleficence (doing no harm), verity (being truthful), and justice (equally distributing resources/care). Ethical conflicts may occur because of differences in cultural and ethical values, but they may also result from decisions that must be made regarding care, such as whether to provide CPR in a wilderness situation when the treatment is likely futile, situations involving triage in which some patients are given priority over others, situations that involve professional misconduct (such as EMS personnel being abusive toward patients), and incidents of patient dumping because the patient has inadequate insurance or an inability to pay. EMS personnel have a moral obligation to make decisions about care in good faith and in the patient's best interest.

DECISION-MAKING MODELS

Do no harm	This model is based on nonmaleficence, the requirement that the treatment provided does no harm; however, by their nature, some treatments can and often do harm patients, so the underlying intent and goal of treatment must be considered when making decisions. For example, CPR may be carried out to save a patient's life and may be done with correct technique but still may result in rib fractures.
In good faith	The motive for a decision should be honest and fair, and decisions should be made with a sincere intention to do good even though the outcome may be negative. For example, EMS personnel may provide a treatment for a patient in good faith although the treatment proves to be ineffective for that particular patient.

| Patient's best interest | Making a decision in the patient's best interest includes considering the patient's or parents' (in the case of children) wishes, the best clinical judgment, the best choice of various options, the chances for improvement/decline, and religious/cultural preferences. |

Anatomy and Physiology

BODY PLANES AND ANATOMIC TERMS

Body planes include the following:

- Sagittal/Lateral: Vertical plane separating right from left.
- Median/Midsagittal: Sagittal plane at the midline (middle) separating the body into equal halves.
- Coronal/Frontal: Vertical plane separating anterior (front) from posterior (back).
- Axial/Transverse: Horizontal plane that separates the body into superior (upper) and inferior (lower) parts.
- A cross section is an axial/transverse (horizontal) cut through a tissue specimen or body structure, whereas a longitudinal section is a sagittal or coronal (vertical) cut.
- Medial is toward the midline, whereas lateral is away from the midline and to the side. Distal is farthest from the point of reference, and proximal is closest. When describing an area of the patient's body, the description should be patient oriented, using phrases such as "patient's left" and "patient's right" to ensure accurate interpretation.

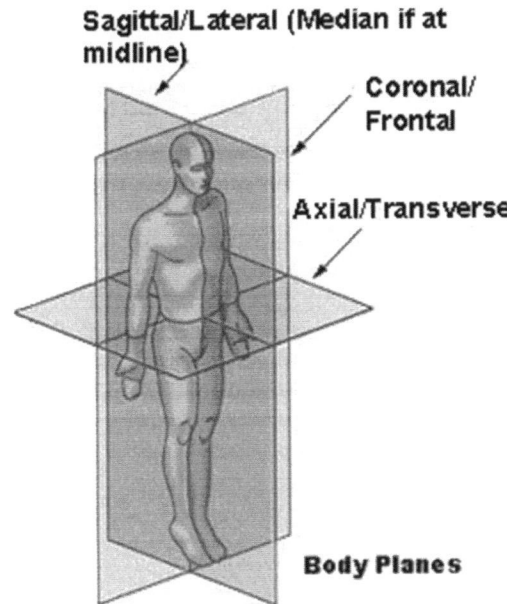

Body Planes

Medical Terminology

COMMON MEDICAL PREFIXES

Term	Meaning	Examples
Cardio-	Heart	Cardiovascular (heart and vessels), cardiology (study of the heart)
Neuro-	Nerves	Neurology (study of the nerves), neuron (nerve cell)
Hyper-	Enlarged, excessive, high	Hypertrophy (enlarged tissue), hyperemesis (excessive vomiting), hyperactive (overactive), hypertension (high BP)
Hypo-	Under, beneath, low	Hypoglycemia (low blood sugar), hypotension (low BP), hypoxia (low oxygen)
Naso-	Nose	Nasopharyngeal (nose and throat), nasal (referring to the nose)
Oro-	Mouth	Oropharyngeal (mouth and throat), oral (referring to the mouth)
Arterio-	Artery	Arteriovenous (artery and vein), arterial (referring to arteries)
Hemo- Hemato-	Blood	Hemolysis (breakdown of blood), hemoglobin (blood component), hematology (study of blood)
Therm-	Temperature	Thermoregulation (temperature regulation), thermometer (temperature measurement)
Vaso-	Vessels	Vasoconstriction (narrowing of vessels), vasodilation (widening of vessels)
Tachy-	Rapid	Tachycardia (rapid heart rate), tachypnea (rapid respirations)
Brady-	Slow	Bradycardia (slow heart rate), bradypnea (slow respirations)

Pathophysiology

Respiratory Compromise

Respiratory compromise may relate to problems with the following:

- Airway: The airway is blocked because of a foreign body, the tongue (especially in unconscious patients and young children), blood or secretions, edema (swelling), or trauma (blunt or penetrating).
- Respirations: The patient is unable to adequately breathe in enough oxygen because of inadequate oxygen in the environment, poison gases (such as carbon monoxide), lung infection (pneumonia), illness that narrows the breathing passages (chronic obstructive pulmonary disease [COPD], bronchitis), excess fluid in the lungs (pulmonary edema), excess fluid between the lung tissue and the blood vessels (leaving inadequate blood volume), and impaired circulation.
- Ventilation: The rate or depth of breathing is inadequate for air exchange; the volume of air breathed in is too small; or air exchange is impaired by altered consciousness, unconsciousness, chest injury, overdose of medication (such as narcotics), poisoning, and disease (such as amyotrophic lateral sclerosis [ALS], sometimes called Lou Gehrig's disease).

Shock

Shock, which is impaired blood flow to the body tissues (cells and organs), may relate to problems with the following:

- Heart: If the heart rate is too slow or too rapid and contractions are ineffectual, insufficient blood is pumped to the lungs for oxygenation and to the cells and body organs. Heart problems may relate to heart disease (such as heart failure), poisoning, and artificial ventilation that is excessive or ineffective.
- Blood vessels: Blood vessels may be unable to constrict, resulting in vasodilation and lowering of the BP. This most often occurs because of cervical (neck) spinal cord injuries, severe infection, or anaphylactic reaction.
- Blood: The volume of circulating blood or blood components may be inadequate to nurture the body cells and organs because of excessive bleeding or vomiting, diarrhea, or burns, which may result in dehydration.

Control of Respirations

The brain's **respiratory center** in the medulla oblongata responds to the body's chemical and mechanical signals. The medulla oblongata contains chemoreceptors that respond to changes in the pH in the fluid surrounding it and the carotid arteries and aorta contain peripheral chemoreceptors that respond to decreases in oxygen and pH. If the blood becomes more acidotic, the medulla oblongata increases the respiratory rate and the tidal volume. If the blood becomes more alkalotic, the medulla oblongata does the opposite in order to maintain the blood pH within the normal range. Mechanical/Stretch receptors are located in the lungs, upper airways, chest wall, and diaphragm, helping to control respirations. The stretch receptors respond when the lungs inflate and send a message to the medulla oblongata via the vagus nerve to prevent overinflation and vice versa. In healthy individuals, increases in carbon dioxide or a decrease in pH cause an increase in the respiratory rate whereas increased oxygen decreases the respiratory rate. In conditions such as COPD in which carbon dioxide is chronically high, this mechanism is impaired.

Ventilation (V)/Perfusion (Q) Ratio and Mismatch

Ventilation (V) and perfusion (Q) are expressed in the ventilation/perfusion ratio (V/Q ratio). Ideally, the volume of blood perfusing the lungs (4–5 L) should equal the volume of gas reaching the alveoli each minute throughout all parts of the lungs, providing a V/Q ratio of 1:1. However, V and Q do not always match, a situation referred to as V/Q mismatch. For example, there is more ventilation than perfusion at the lung apices and less ventilation than perfusion at the lung bases. Additionally, some diseases and conditions may cause

V/Q mismatch, such as COPD, severe asthma, pneumonia, pulmonary embolism, and atelectasis. Ventilation may be limited (such as with asthma) while perfusion remains stable, resulting in hypoxemia because of an inadequate intake of oxygen. A pulmonary embolus or other disease may block an area of the lung so that ventilation is adequate but perfusion is impaired, again resulting in hypoxemia.

Myocardial Effectiveness

Myocardial effectiveness depends on cardiac output, the volume of blood pumped from the left ventricle of the heart in one minute, and it equals the stroke volume (the volume of blood ejected with each ventricular contraction, usually about 70 mL in an adult) times the heart rate. So, if the heart rate is 60, the cardiac output (60 × 70) would be 4200 mL (normally 4–8 L/min). Stroke volume is determined by the following factors:

- Preload: Stretch/Tension of muscle fibers, usually corresponding to the end-diastolic pressure when the ventricles are filled.
- Afterload: The amount of pressure that the ventricles must work against when ejecting blood during systole, representing the systemic vascular resistance.
- Myocardial contractility: The amount of stretch in the myocardial muscle fibers, which determines the forcefulness of the contractions.

Systemic vascular resistance increases when vessels constrict and decreases when they dilate. With atherosclerosis, the vessels become more rigid and the lumen (opening) tends to narrow from plaque deposits, increasing systemic vascular resistance and increasing the burden on the heart.

Blood Pressure (BP)

Blood pressure (BP; the force of the blood against the vessel walls) is necessary to maintain adequate perfusion. BP relates to cardiac output (CO) and systemic vascular resistance (SVR) (aka total peripheral resistance). SVR results from the resistance of the blood flow from the lumen (opening) of the vessel and the viscosity of the blood. The mechanisms that control BP affect either the CO or the SVR. If the CO remains stable but the SVR increases, then the BP rises. Although the stroke volume often varies little, the heart rate can increase markedly, affecting cardiac output. As the CO increases, the BP increases. If the CO decreases, then the BP decreases as well. As the SVR increases, the BP increases; and as the SVR decreases, the BP decreases. The body responds to changes in CO, SVR, and BP through vasoconstriction, which increases the SVR and BP, and vasodilation, which decreases the SVR and BP. Thus, if a patient is in shock and the CO and BP fall, the body reacts with vasoconstriction to increase the BP.

Life Span Development

Normal Vital Signs from Neonate to Older Adulthood

Age	Heart rate	Respirations	BP (mm Hg)
Neonate (newborn)	100–220 (average 140–160) begins to slow after 3 months	40–60 for a few minutes, then 30–40	Systolic 70–90
Toddler (12–36 mos.)	80–130	20–30	Systolic 70–100
Preschool (3 to 5)	80–120	20–30	Systolic 80–110
School age (6-12)	70–110	20–30	80–120/60–80
Adolescence (13–18)	55–100	12–20	110–131/64–84
Early adulthood (19–40)	60–100 (average 80)	12–20	100–119/60–79 to 140/90 (high)
Middle adulthood (41–60)	60–100 (average 80)	12–20	100–119/60–79 to 140/90 (high)
Late adulthood (61+)	60–100 (average 70)	12–20	100–119/60–79 to 140/90 (high)

Levels of Disease Prevention

Levels of disease prevention include the following:

- Primary: The goal is to prevent the initial occurrence of a health problem, such as a disease or injury, through activities such as immunizations, smoking cessation, fluoride supplementation of water, promotion of seat belt and helmet use, and use of child car seat restraints. Interventions are often aimed at the general public or large groups of people.
- Secondary: The goal is to identify diseases or conditions quickly and provide prompt intervention to provide treatment and prevent further disability through activities such as BP screenings, breast and testicular self-examinations, hearing and vision screenings, mammography, and pregnancy testing.
- Tertiary: The goal is to assist those who already have disease or disability to prevent further progress of the disease and to allow people to achieve the maximum quality of life through activities such as support groups, counseling, diet and exercise, stress management, and supportive services.

Public Health

PUBLIC HEALTH SYSTEM

EMS are part of the **public health system**, a network of private, nonprofit, and government agencies and healthcare providers providing public health services in a wide range of areas. The primary services provided by the public health system include the following:

- Monitoring community health.
- Identifying hazards to health in the environment/community.
- Educating people about health issues.
- Mobilizing various agencies and individuals to take action.
- Enforcing public safety laws/regulations.
- Ensuring that healthcare providers are qualified, licensed, and certified as required.
- Ensuring that health care is available.
- Assessing the effectiveness of health care.
- Researching health problems and finding solutions.

Public health laws/regulations may be federal, state, or tribal and cover issues such as immunization requirements, drinking water/sewage system standards, air quality, water fluoridation, restrictions on tobacco use (age and place), restrictions on drinking (age, driving), speed limits, prenatal care, abuse (child, older adult, sexual, and domestic), safety equipment, and safe lifting. Healthy People 2020, of the US Department of Health and Human Services, provides goals and objectives for health-related public policies.

SAFETY EQUIPMENT AND EDUCATION

Safety equipment may include a wide variety of devices, including smoke alarms and carbon monoxide alarms. Some safety equipment protects people from falls, especially older adults. These may include safety rails, grab bars, canes, and walkers. EMS personnel are often involved in public education regarding the following:

- <u>Car seats:</u> Should be properly secured in the backseat of a motor vehicle. They should be rear facing for infants and toddlers up to 2 years of age (or the maximum recommended height and weight) and forward-facing with a harness for toddlers and preschoolers. School-aged children should use booster seats with a belt and harness until they are at least 4 feet 9 inches tall. Children younger than age 13 should not ride in a front seat.
- <u>Seat belts:</u> All people in a motor vehicle should be secured with seat belts and shoulder harnesses.
- <u>Helmets:</u> Should fit properly and snugly, cover the top of the forehead, and have a securing chinstrap. They should be worn when riding a bicycle or motorcycle and engaging in sports activities such as rollerblading but not on playground equipment or when climbing trees.

Pharmacology

PHARMACODYNAMICS AND PHARMACOKINETICS

Pharmacodynamics relates to biological effects (therapeutic or adverse) of drug administration. Responses may be continuous, such as BP variations, or dichotomous, in which an event either occurs or does not (such as recovery). Information from pharmacodynamics provides feedback to modify medication dosage (pharmacokinetics). **Pharmacokinetics** relates to the route of administration, the absorption, the dosage, the frequency of administration, the distribution, and the serum levels achieved over time. Most drugs are cleared through the kidneys. Elimination half-time is the time needed to reduce plasma concentrations to 50% during elimination. Age and weight may impact the absorption and elimination of drugs. Drugs have a generic/scientific/nonproprietary name (acetaminophen) and a brand/trade/proprietary name (Tylenol). Emergency medications include solids (pills, capsules, powders), liquids (enteral [ingested] or parenteral [injected]), and gases (inhaled). Enteral medications may be given orally (glucose) or sublingually (nitroglycerin). Parenteral drugs are inhaled (oxygen, albuterol) or injected (epinephrine).

COMMONLY ADMINISTERED MEDICATIONS

Medication	Dose/Route/Use	Side effects/Interactions
Aspirin	Orally, 325 mg, chew and swallow for fast action when having a heart attack.	Avoid with signs of stroke or gastrointestinal (GI) bleeding. Decreases clotting time and may increase the risk of bleeding.
Glucose	Orally for hypoglycemia. May be in liquid or tablet form, or a glass of orange juice may be given.	Minimal unless hyperglycemic.
Oxygen	Inhaled, usually 2–6 L, but it varies according to protocol.	Minimal, although oxygen toxicity can occur with high doses for prolonged periods of time.
Bronchodilators (albuterol, levalbuterol)	Inhaled, usually two puffs of a handheld inhaler. Dosage varies according to the medication. For bronchospasm, wheezing.	Adverse effects: tachycardia, dizziness, nervousness, tremor, headache, rhinitis, increased cough.
Epinephrine (EpiPen)	Autoinjector, 0.3 mg 1:1000 for ≥66 lb. 0.15 mg 1:2000 for 33–66 lb. for severe allergic reaction/anaphylaxis.	Avoid using with antihistamines, thyroid hormones, and alpha blockers. Adverse effects: drowsiness, headache, palpitations, nervousness, tremors.
Nitroglycerin	Sublingually for angina (chest pain), 0.3–0.6 mg, repeated every 5 minutes up to three times.	Avoid with myocardial infarction. Adverse effects: headache, flushing, dizziness, orthostatic hypotension, palpitations. Interactions: Avoid with erectile dysfunction drugs (sildenafil, tadalafil, vardenafil).

DRUG DOSE CALCULATIONS

Desired dose and volume/concentration on hand	Milligrams (mg) needed/mg available in dose × volume per dose = current dose.	If an infant is to receive 65 mg of acetaminophen elixir that contains 80 mg per 5 milliliters (mL): 65 mg/80 mg = 0.8125 ×5 = 4.06 = 4 mL.
Convert pounds (lb) to kilograms (kg)	No. of lb/2.2 kg.	Infant weight 16 lb.: 16/2.2 = 7.3 kg, rounded to 7 kg.

IV flow rate in drops per minute	Volume (mL)/time (minutes) × drop factor = flow rate. Note: The standard drop factor is 15 drops/mL, but microdrip infusion sets (used with pediatrics or small volumes) have 60 drops/mL.	If a patient is to receive 1200 mL of 5% dextrose in water (D5W) in 5 hours (300 minutes) and the drop factor of the infusion set is 15 drops per mL: 1000/300 × 15 = 49.9 = 50 drops/min.

MEDICATION LEGISLATION

Act/Agency	Purpose
Pure Food and Drug Act (1906)	Consumer protection act intended to prevent the manufacture, sale, and transportation of adulterated foods, drugs, and alcoholic beverages.
Federal Food, Drug, and Cosmetic Act (1938)	Provides authority to the FDA to oversee food, drug, and cosmetic safety.
Harrison Narcotics Tax Act (1914)	Provides authority for regulation and taxation of production, importation, and distribution of coca/opium products, such as narcotics.
Controlled Substances Act (1970)	Establishes US drug policy and five schedules under which drugs are classified, implemented by the DEA and the FDA.
Food and Drug Administration (FDA)	Consumer protection agency that protects public health through the control and supervision of drugs, vaccines, blood transfusions, medical devices, cosmetics, foods, tobacco, and dietary supplements.
Drug Enforcement Agency (DEA)	Law enforcement agency, part of the Department of Justice, enforces the Controlled Substances Act and combats drug smuggling/use.

ASSISTANCE WITH MEDICATIONS AND THE FIVE RIGHTS OF MEDICATION ADMINISTRATION

The AEMT may assist patients to self-administer medications or administer them directly depending on the scope of practice and protocols. Medical direction may be offline, which means standing orders are available to treat specific conditions or written protocols have been established that must be followed. online medical direction requires verbal contact with a medical director. When receiving an online medication order, the AEMT should use the echo technique (repeating back the orders to ensure that they were understood correctly) and clarify any orders that are confusing or unclear.

The **five rights of medication administration** include the following:

1. Right patient: The medication should be prescribed specifically for that patient.
2. Right medication: Correct choice for the patient's condition, and it matches the prescription.
3. Right route: Appropriate for the patient's condition, enteral or parenteral.
4. Right dose: As prescribed and appropriate for the patient's age, weight, and condition.
5. Right time: The medication is not expired, and it is administered at the time ordered, such as "stat" (immediately) or "every 5 minutes × 3."

Airway Management, Respirations and Artificial Ventilation

RESPIRATORY (AIRWAY) SYSTEM

Air enters the **respiratory system** through the nose and mouth, where it is warmed and moistened, and it passes through the pharynx (back of throat) and the larynx (voice box) into the trachea (windpipe). The epiglottis is a cartilage flap that closes over the larynx when swallowing so food enters the esophagus (the tube leading to the stomach). The trachea branches into the right and left bronchi (large tubes) that carry the air into the lungs. Each bronchus branches into smaller bronchioles and millions of alveoli (small air sacs), which are covered with webs of tiny capillaries that deliver carbon dioxide and pick up oxygen (external respiration). The muscles of respiration are the diaphragm and the intercostal muscles (between the ribs), but accessory muscles in the neck and collarbone area may help during respiratory distress. The heart circulates unoxygenated blood to the lungs. After oxygenation, the blood returns to the heart and into the general circulation and body cells where gas exchange occurs again (internal respiration). Cells intake oxygen and nutrients and release carbon dioxide and waste products (cellular respiration).

Pediatrics: Infants are obligate nasal breathers for the first two to four months and usually only breathe through the nose, although they can generally breathe through the mouth if necessary. However, if nasal passages are blocked, they may quickly develop respiratory distress. Chest wall compliance is greater in infants and small children, so they must work harder than an adult to move the same amount of air. Additionally, proportionally the airway is smaller, the tongue is larger, and the cartilage is softer, increasing the risk of obstruction.

Older adults: Breathing capacity tends to decline after age 40 because the number of alveoli decreases and the size of alveoli increases, resulting in less surface for and less efficient gas exchange. Lung elasticity also decreases, resulting in decreased vital capacity. The chest muscles tend to weaken and stiffen with age, and older adults have a lowered ability to cough and clear the airways.

> **Review Video: Respiratory System**
> Visit mometrix.com/academy and enter code: 783075

LIFE SUPPORT CHAIN

Critical to the **life support chain** are oxygenation and perfusion. Oxygenation involves gas exchange of carbon dioxide for oxygen at the alveolar/capillary level and the cell/capillary level. Perfusion involves the transport of blood, which carries oxygen, glucose, and other nutrients as well as waste products throughout the body. Oxygen and glucose are essential for cell functioning. Glucose is produced by the digestion of carbohydrates (starches); it is the primary energy source for the body; and its use is controlled by insulin, which is produced by the pancreas. Excess glucose is stored in the liver as glycogen for later use or is converted to fat. These fundamental elements are affected by the composition of ambient air (usually 21% oxygen), airway patency, ventilation, regulation of respiration, blood volume and transport, heart action, and blood vessel size and resistance.

PHYSIOLOGY OF RESPIRATION

The **physiology of respiration** includes the following:

- Ventilation: Movement of air in and out of the lungs during inhalation and exhalation. The normal tidal volume (air exchange when breathing normally) for an adult is about 500 mL, but it is lower for infants and children (5–7 mL/kg for neonates, 6–8 mL/kg for children). Breathing may be impaired by disease (muscular dystrophy), drugs, trauma, bronchoconstriction, allergic reactions, foreign body obstructions, and infection.
- Oxygenation: The process by which oxygen molecules bind to hemoglobin in the blood. The blood saturation level reflects the amount of oxygen that is dissolved in the blood and available to body tissues, and it should be ≥95%.
- Respiration: The process by which the lungs exchange carbon dioxide for oxygen in the alveoli and provide this oxygenated blood to body tissues. Respiration may be external (inspiration, expiration), internal (exchange of gas), or cellular (cells perform tasks that require oxygen and glucose [sugar] and produce carbon dioxide as a waste product). Respiration may be impaired by a lack of air, toxins/poisons, and ineffective circulation (shock, cardiac arrest).

Tidal volume	Normal volume of gas inhaled during one respiration cycle (approximately 500 mL in a healthy adult).
Inspiratory reserve volume	Volume of air inhaled greater than the tidal volume during forced deep inhalation (up to 3000 mL).
Dead space	Volume of inhaled gas that does not take part in gas exchange.
Alveolar dead space	Volume of alveoli that are ventilated but not perfused.
Vital capacity	Maximum volume of gas that can be forcefully exhaled from the lungs following a full inhalation.
Minute volume	Volume of gas expelled from the lungs in one minute (the respiratory rate × the tidal volume).
Residual volume	Volume of gas remaining in the lungs after one full, forced exhalation.
Total lung capacity	Vital capacity plus residual volume; it is the total volume that the lungs can contain (usually about 6000 mL for adults).
Cellular respiration	Use of oxygen and glucose to produce energy at the cellular level and the creation of water and carbon dioxide as by-products of metabolism.
Oxygenation	Process by which oxygen molecules bind to hemoglobin in the blood.

AIRWAY ASSESSMENT AND MANUAL MEASURES TO CLEAR THE AIRWAY

Indications of an adequate airway include a normal voice and speaking ability and audible and visible air exchange. Indications of inadequate airway include unusual breathing sounds (wheezing, stridor), hoarse voice/inability to speak, and no audible or visible air exchange. Airway obstruction may result from the tongue falling back, food, a foreign body, vomit, blood, teeth, and edema (swelling). **Maneuvers** include the following:

- Head tilt/chin lift: Hyperextend the neck by tilting the patient's head back with one hand on his or her forehead to straighten the airway and lift the tongue. Then lift the chin and pull forward with the fingers of the other hand under the chin with the thumb on top. The chin lift pulls the mandible (jaw) forward. This prevents the tongue from blocking the pharynx. Contraindications to the head tilt/chin lift include suspected cervical spine and neck injuries.
- Jaw thrust: This technique is used with a suspected spinal cord or neck injury in which extending the neck must be avoided. From behind, place the fingers behind the angles of the patient's lower jaw and place your thumbs on the chin; move the jaw upward until it is extended while using the thumbs to slightly open the patient's mouth. Contraindications include severe facial injuries.

- Modified chin lift/jaw thrust: This technique is used with a suspected spinal cord/neck injury with an unstable cervical spine. From the head of the patient, place your thumbs on his or her cheekbones and place your fingers under the patient's mandible, and then pull the mandible upward with the fingers while applying pressure with the thumbs. If using a mask for ventilation, place the mask in position and secure it with your thumbs while your fingers thrust the patient's jaw forward.

VENTILATION

Ventilation is adequate if the respiratory rate, depth of respiration, and effort of breathing are normal. Signs of inadequate ventilation include the following:

- Increased effort of breathing: Nasal flaring, sternal retraction (infants), use of abdominal or intercostal (between the ribs) muscles, sweating, sitting in the tripod position (upright, leaning forward, hands on knees).
- Abnormal breath sounds: Wheezes, rales (crackles), and/or rhonchi (snoring/whistling sounds).
- Abnormal depth of breathing: Hypoventilation (too shallow) or hyperventilation (too deep).
- Abnormal rate of breathing: Tachypnea (too fast) or bradypnea (too slow).
- Abnormal chest wall movement: Splinting, asymmetric, paradoxical (chest wall/diaphragm move in during inhalation and out during exhalation—opposite of normal).
- Irregular breathing pattern: May include periods of apnea (no breathing).

Patients with inadequate ventilation or apnea in which there is no breathing or only occasional gasping require ventilation assistance, such as with a pocket mask or bag-valve mask (BVM).

OROPHARYNGEAL AIRWAY (OPA)

The **oropharyngeal airway** (OPA), a blind-insertion airway device, may be inserted to provide better ventilation, but the OPA requires the head tilt/chin lift or modified jaw thrust as well because the device alone does not ensure a patent airway. The OPA is indicated for unconscious patients, patients with no gag reflex, and patients who are apneic (not breathing) and require ventilatory aid. The OPA is often inserted if a patient stops breathing, such as with a cardiac arrest. The OPA is contraindicated in conscious patients and those with a gag reflex. To insert the OPA, perform the following steps:

- Estimate the length of the OPA by measuring the patient from the angle of the jaw or the tip of the earlobe to the corner of the mouth.
- Select the correct size.
- Open the patient's mouth using the cross-finger technique. Suction any secretions.
- Tilt the head back (if possible). Insert the device with the tip of the OPA pointing upward for adults and downward for children.
- Rotate the OPA into position for adults.
- Ensure that the phalanges of the mouthpiece are securely against the patient's mouth.
- Check to make sure the OPA is patent (open).

NASOPHARYNGEAL AIRWAY (NPA)

The **nasopharyngeal airway** (NPA), a blind-insertion airway device, is indicated for unconscious or semiconscious patients who still have a gag reflex or those who cannot tolerate an oropharyngeal airway (OPA), but it should be avoided with severe head injury, risk of basal skull fracture, nasal bleeding, and history of deviated septum or nasal fracture. It's important to use the appropriate size. To insert the NPA, perform the following steps: Choose a size that is slightly smaller in diameter than the patient's nostril. Measure from the tip of the earlobe to the tip of the nose. Lubricate the NPA with water-soluble lubricant and insert it in the larger and most patent (open) nostril. If inserting into the right nostril, insert with the bevel (tip) angled toward the nasal septum (the bony cartilage division between the nostrils). If inserting it into the left nostril, invert the NPA to angle the bevel toward the septum. When the NPA reaches the throat, rotate it 180° into the proper position.

Bag-Valve Mask (BVM)

Bag-valve mask (BVM) ventilation equipment used for positive-pressure ventilation (PPV) includes a mask, a ventilator bag, an oxygen reservoir bag, and an attachment for oxygen delivery. The correct mask size is important: The mask should not cover the chin. BVM is contraindicated if the airway is not patent, but it is used for abnormal breathing and for respiratory distress/failure. BVM requires two EMS personnel—one to control the mask and the other to control the bag. Steps are as follows:

- Position yourself behind the patient's head, place the mask over the patient's nose and mouth, and make a tight seal by holding it in place with your thumbs and index fingers while your other fingers slide under the patient's jaw to lift the chin.
- Squeeze the bag with inhalations initially for 5 to 10 breaths and then adjust the rate to at least 12 breaths per minute, slowly adjusting the rate and tidal volume delivered.

Assessment of lung compliance (the ability to expand and contract) includes observation of chest movement, rate of respirations, and the feel of BVM. Difficult ventilation suggests impaired compliance. Note: The BVM can be used with or without oxygen.

Laryngeal-Mask Airway (LMA)

The laryngeal-mask airway (LMA), a blind-insertion airway device, is an intermediate airway allowing ventilation but not complete respiratory control. The LMA consists of an inflatable cuff (mask) with a connecting tube. It may be used when tracheal intubation can't be done or as a conduit for later blind insertion of an endotracheal tube. The head and neck must be in a neutral position for insertion. If the patient has a gag reflex, then conscious sedation or topical anesthesia (deep oropharyngeal) is required. The LMA is inserted by sliding the airway along the hard palate, using the finger as a guide, into the pharynx, and the ring is inflated to create a seal around the opening to the larynx, allowing ventilation with mild positive pressure. The LMA ProSeal has a modified cuff that extends onto the back of the mask to improve the seal. The CobraPLA (perilaryngeal airway) has a larger pharyngeal cuff and provides a better seal. The LMA is contraindicated in morbid obesity, with obstructions or abnormalities of the oropharynx, and in nonfasting patients because some aspiration is still possible.

Esophageal Tracheal Combitube (ETC)

The **esophageal tracheal Combitube (ETC)** is a blind-insertion airway device and an intermediate airway that contains two lumens (channels). It can be inserted into either the trachea or the esophagus ($\leq 91\%$). The twin-lumen tube has a proximal cuff providing a seal for the oropharynx and a distal cuff providing a seal around the distal tube. Prior to insertion, the Combitube cuffs should be checked for leaks (with 15 mL of air into the distal cuff and 85 mL of air into the proximal cuff). The patient should be nonresponsive and with no gag reflex with his or her head in a neutral position. The tube is passed along the tongue and into the pharynx, using markings on the tube (black guidelines) to determine the depth by aligning the ETC with the upper incisors or the alveolar ridge. Once in place, the distal cuff is inflated (10–15 mL) and then placement in the trachea or esophagus should be determined so the proper lumen for ventilation can be used. The proximal cuff is inflated (usually to 50–75 mL) and ventilation is started. A capnogram should be used to confirm ventilation.

Tracheostomy Care

A **tracheostomy** is a surgical opening (stoma) into the trachea to form an airway in cases of upper respiratory obstruction or long-term mechanical ventilation. Tubes are inserted into the opening to provide a conduit and maintain the opening. Tracheostomy tubes are usually metal or plastic—most are now lacking an inner cannula because they are nonadherent—and secured with ties around the neck. Tracheostomy tubes are changed using clean technique. For tracheostomy care, place the patient in the semi-Fowler's position and don PPE. Unlock and remove the inner cannula if present, clean with a 3% hydrogen peroxide, and rinse with sterile water. Wipe the area around the stoma with sterile water. If changing the outer cannula, remove the tube and clean it, then reinsert it at a 45° angle to the throat. If suctioning, preoxygenate, set the pressure to 120 to 150 mm Hg, and use sterile technique, inserting the catheter 0.5 cm longer than the length of the tracheostomy tube. Suction only on withdrawal for no more than 10 seconds. If repeating, oxygenate for 3–4 breaths between.

Sellick's Maneuver (Cricoid Pressure)

Sellick's maneuver (cricoid pressure) may be used with PPV to prevent air from flowing down the esophagus and into the stomach rather than down the trachea and into the lungs because stomach distension increases the risk of vomiting. This maneuver may also be used with intubation to prevent regurgitation of stomach contents and aspiration. Sellick's maneuver may be used on unconscious patients receiving a mask or BVM. The procedure consists of applying pressure downward to the cricoid cartilage of the neck (which is at the bottom of the larynx and blocks the upper esophagus) with the thumb and index finger. Pressure is usually applied at 30 to 40 newtons but no greater than 40 newtons because too great of force may block the airway. The maneuver may also cause nausea and vomiting and, with severe pressure, may result in rupture of the esophagus. Vomiting is a contraindication.

Normal Negative-Pressure Breathing and Positive-Pressure Breathing

Negative-pressure breathing (normal)	Positive-pressure breathing
The movement downward of the diaphragm (triggered by the phrenic nerves) creates a negative pressure in the lungs, drawing air into them. Blood flows from the lungs to the heart and back and to the body at a steady rate in normal breathing. The epiglottis closes the esophagus during inhalation, preventing air from entering the stomach.	Ventilation forces air into the lungs, and this can result in dysfunction of the diaphragm because it is responding to a change in pressure rather than stimulation by the phrenic nerve. Blood flow from the lungs is reduced, resulting in decreased cardiac (heart) output. The epiglottis may stay open during ventilation, allowing air into the stomach and increasing the risk of vomiting.

Recovery Position

The **recovery position** is used for patients who are unconscious but breathing (such as those with a drug overdose or after a seizure) and have no life-threatening injuries. This position helps to maintain a patent airway and reduces the risk of aspiration from vomitus.

	Kneeling beside the patient, lift his or her chin to ensure that the airway is open and place his or her closest arm at right angle to body with hand up. Place the patient's farthest arm around his or her neck with the hand touching the opposite cheek. Flex the patient's knee to 90° until the foot is flat on the floor/surface.
	Using the patient's knee as a fulcrum and supporting the farthest arm and shoulder, roll the patient onto his or her side by pulling on the farthest knee. Make sure that the top knee contacts the floor/surface to support the patient's body and that the top hand is under his or her head to keep the neck in a neutral position.

Upper Airway Suctioning

Suctioning devices may be vehicle mounted or portable and should be checked to ensure that the tubing is intact and the canister has an airtight seal. Patients at risk for aspiration include those with an altered level of consciousness, those having difficulty swallowing or breathing, trauma patients, obese patients, and those with recurrent vomiting. Oral suctioning is used to remove secretions, vomitus, and blood. Suctioning may be done with a rigid-tip catheter (Yankauer) or a soft-tip catheter. Techniques include the following:

- Don a mask and gloves.
- Measure the patient from the tip of the ear to the corner of the mouth to determine how far to insert the catheter.
- Turn on the suction.
- Use the cross-finger technique to open the mouth.
- Insert the tube and apply suction. The rigid catheter has a finger control to start and stop suction.
- Move the catheter around the gum line and over the tongue to the back of the mouth, but avoid stimulating the gag reflex.
- Suction for no longer than 15 seconds at a time.
- Note: Clear a small infant's airway by suctioning the nose with a bulb syringe.

PORTABLE OXYGEN CYLINDERS

Two commonly used sizes of **portable oxygen cylinders** are D tanks (M15; 350 L) and E tanks (M24; 625 L). The AEMT should use protective equipment (goggles, gloves). The cylinder should be placed upright. A label over the holes on the top of the cylinder indicates that the cylinder is full. Remove the label, leaving the washers in place unless the washers are built into the regulator. Face the opening of the tank away, and use the key to crack the cylinder by letting out a small amount of oxygen. Apply the regulator and slide it into place. Tighten and then open the cylinder to check for pressure (there should be at least 200 psi). Close the cylinder, attach the oxygen tubing to the regulator, set the oxygen flow to the correct amount of liters, and then open the cylinder and administer oxygen to the patient. When discontinuing use of the cylinder, turn off the cylinder, remove the oxygen tubing, turn the oxygen flow setting up to bleed air from the regular, and remove the regulator.

ASSESSMENT OF OXYGENATION

Assessment of oxygenation includes the following:

- Evaluate respirations: Note the signs of respiratory distress—rapid breathing, slow breathing, use of accessory muscles, nasal flaring, and sternal retraction—because they may indicate inadequate oxygenation.
- Assess mental status: Confusion may be associated with hypo-oxygenation (low oxygen), but it's important to determine a baseline mental status if possible because the patient may have dementia or may be confused because of medications.
- Assess skin: Note cyanosis (blue tinge) especially around the mouth, fingertips, and oral mucous membranes because this indicates a lack of oxygen. Another sign is pallor. Mottling of the skin, purplish or reddish discoloration especially on the knees and feet, indicates hypo-oxygenation and is a common indication that death is near.
- Monitor pulse oximetry: It should be 95%–100%. If a patient has mild respiratory disease, the pulse oximetry level may be as low as 90% and still be within the normal range for the patient. Readings less than 90%–92% indicate hypoxemia (low oxygen in the blood).

ASSESSMENT OF RESPIRATIONS AND SUPPLEMENTAL OXYGEN ADMINISTRATION

When **assessing respirations**, the AEMT should note the patient's gag reflex and rate of respirations (whether it is normal for the patient's age or it is too fast, too slow, or absent). The AEMT should also evaluate the rise and fall of the chest and any abnormal movements (such as sternal retraction, nasal flaring) noisy breathing (gurgling, wheezing), the use of accessory muscles, or the tripod position (sitting, leaning forward, and supporting the body with the hands). If breathing is abnormal or the pulse oximetry is less than 95%, the AEMT should take precautions against bloodstream infection (BSI) and administer **supplemental oxygen** with a nonrebreather mask with the oxygen set at 12–15 L. The reservoir bag of the mask must be completely filled before applying the mask to the patient, securing it with an elastic band about the head. If the patient cannot tolerate the nonrebreather mask, then a nasal cannula may be used with the oxygen flow set at 4–6 L, the prongs inserted into the nostrils, and tubing secured by looping over the ears and tightening under the chin.

PULSE OXIMETRY

Pulse oximetry uses an external oximeter that attaches to the patient's finger or earlobe to measure arterial oxygen saturation (SPO_2), the percentage of hemoglobin that is saturated with oxygen. The oximeter uses light waves to determine SPO_2. Oxygen saturation should be maintained >95%, although some patients with chronic respiratory disorders, such as COPD, may have lower SPO_2 readings. Results may be compromised by impaired circulation, excessive light, poor positioning, and nail polish. If the SPO_2 reading falls, the oximeter should be repositioned because incorrect positioning is a common cause of inaccurate readings. Oximetry is used for monitoring when patients are on oxygen or mechanical ventilation. Oximeters do not provide information about carbon dioxide levels, so they cannot monitor carbon dioxide retention. Oximeters also cannot differentiate between different forms of hemoglobin, so if the hemoglobin has picked up carbon monoxide, the oximeter will not recognize that.

OXYGEN DELIVERY DEVICES

Oxygen delivery devices provide oxygen-enriched air. Ambient air is about 21% oxygen, so the fraction of inspired air (FIO_2) is 21%.

Oxygen delivery devices	
Nasal cannula (prongs)	FIO_2 of 24%–40% with flows of ≤6 liters per minute (LPM). Humidification should be used for prolonged flow rates of >4 LPM.
Partial rebreather face mask	This mask covers the nose and mouth, delivering FIO_2 of 30%–60%, but the flow of oxygen should be maintained between 6 and 12 LPM to decrease the risk of rebreathing. Because of the higher flow rate, humidification should be used.
Venturi mask	Oxygen entrainment masks come with different-sized color-coded nozzles to more accurately control FIO_2, with different sizes providing different FIO_2 levels, usually ranging from 24% to 50%, although an FIO_2 reading of >35% is not always reliable. The flow rate is 12–15 LPM. Humidifiers may be used.
Non-rebreather mask	This mask covers the mouth and nose with a reservoir bag of oxygen. A one-way valve prevents the patient from rebreathing exhaled air. FIO_2 is about 60%–80% or greater at a flow rate of 15 LPM.

POSITIVE AIRWAY PRESSURE (PAP) DEVICES

All **positive airway pressure** (PAP) devices, such as continuous positive airway pressure (CPAP), have an air blower that delivers pressurized room air to an interface/mask. Pressure can be increased or decreased by adjusting the speed or the amount of airflow, with most machines generating from 2 to 20 cm of water pressure. Carbon dioxide is expelled through a vent or a nonrebreather valve on expiration. Bilevel PAP (BiPAP, BPAP) devices deliver two levels of pressure, which can be preset. Inspiratory PAP (IPAP) is set at a higher level (10 cm H_2O) than is expiratory PAP (EPAP) (5 cm H_2O) to allow a higher pressure needed to open the airway during inspiration but reduce the pressure to facilitate expiration. PAP is indicated for pulmonary edema, CHF, COPD, asthma, and near drowning.

The procedure includes the following:

- Fill the humidifier with distilled water.
- Program the settings.
- Fit the mask and headgear/straps.

- Begin with the pressure at the lowest setting, usually 5 cm H_2O (CPAP), and increase it slowly at 1 cm H_2O every few minutes until the optimal level is reached.
- Monitor the oxygen saturation and respirations.

POCKET-MASK VENTILATION

Pocket-mask ventilation is used when administering cardiopulmonary resuscitation (CPR) to a patient who is in cardiac arrest and apneic (not breathing). If two EMS personnel are available, one should be positioned at the patient's head to administer pocket-mask ventilation while the other does compressions. If there is only one EMS personnel, then that person should be positioned at the patient's side. Administration is as follows:

- Remove the mask from the container and push the flattened mask to open it.
- Wipe the patient's face clean with alcohol swab if necessary to remove secretions, vomitus.
- Do a chin tilt or jaw thrust and place the mask over the patient's nose and mouth, holding it in place with both hands to seal it tightly.
- Take a deep breath and blow in through the one-way valve, watching the chest rise to ensure that ventilation has occurred.
- Continue to ventilate the patient at a rate of 30 compressions to 2 ventilations for CPR.
- Attach supplemental oxygen if available to improve oxygenation.
- Upon patient recovery or completion of CPR, remove the mask, discard the valve, and disinfect the mask.

POSITIVE END-EXPIRATORY PRESSURE (PEEP)

Positive end-expiratory pressure (PEEP) is a setting in mechanical ventilation, that is, the airway pressure at the end of an exhalation. The primary purpose of PEEP is to improve oxygenation by preventing airway collapse. The usual settings are 5 to 25 cm H_2O. PEEP is indicated for respiratory distress syndromes/acute lung injury, pulmonary edema, atelectasis, and severe pneumonia resulting in hypoxemia. PEEP may improve gas exchange and lung compliance and prevent alveolar collapse, but it may also decrease gas exchange and cardiac output and cause hypotension and hypoperfusion of internal organs as well as barotrauma and increased intracranial pressure. PEEP is contraindicated with increased intracranial pressure, low cardiac output, pneumothorax (without a pleural catheter), and hypovolemia. The procedure is as follows:

- Start the setting at 5 cm H_2O, and increase it by 2–3 cm H_2O (not to exceed 15) every 30 to 60 minutes to achieve oxygen saturation of greater than 88% or PaO_2 of greater than 55 mm Hg.

Assessment

PRIMARY ASSESSMENT

After surveying the environment for safety issues, the AEMT should quickly conduct a **primary assessment** to identify conditions that are life-threatening, as follows:

- Level of consciousness: Alert, responsive to verbal stimuli, responsive to painful stimuli, nonresponsive.
- Breathing status: Normal, abnormal, rate abnormalities (>24 or <8), apnea, choking, normal or abnormal chest movement, chest rise and fall, noisy respirations, use of accessory muscles, tripod position, nasal flaring.
- Circulatory status: Radial, carotid pulse, pulse abnormalities, major bleeding, skin color—pink, blue (cyanotic), pale, skin temperature, skin moisture, capillary refill, signs of shock.

Life-threatening conditions must be treated immediately, as follows:

- If there is no radial pulse but there is a carotid pulse, lie the patient flat and elevate his or her feet 8 to 12 inches.
- No pulse: Begin CPR.
- Shock: Lay the patient flat, elevate his or her feet 8–12 inches, and administer oxygen at 15 L/min.
- Bleeding: Apply pressure to control any bleeding.
- Abnormal breathing: Provide oxygen with a nonrebreather mask. If the patient is unresponsive, cyanotic, or in respiratory distress, use a BVM with supplemental oxygen.
- Unresponsive: Ensure a patent airway.

Based on the assessment, the patient is classified as stable, potentially unstable, or unstable.

HISTORY TAKING ON ARRIVAL AT A SCENE

History taking should include the following:

- Chief complaint: If the patient is unable to explain, information may be gathered from his or her family, friends, or others who are present. Look for a medical alert bracelet or other such jewelry.
- Nature of the illness or mechanism of injury: Reason for calling EMS, cause of injury, type of illness. Look for environmental clues (fire, drug paraphernalia, motor vehicle accident).
- Signs and symptoms observed or reported by the patient: Skin temperature, open wounds, BP abnormalities, pain, or difficulty breathing.
- Precipitating events: Falls, accidents, violence, eating, exercising, walking, driving.
- Pediatric considerations: Check capillary refill to assess blood flow in infants and children younger than 6. Assess the pulse at the brachial artery (inside of the upper arm) for infants up to 1 year of age and the carotid artery in the neck for children older than 1 year. May need to use distraction to gain trust and alleviate fear. Encourage the parents/caregivers to hold the child if possible and assist in calming the child.
- Geriatric (older adult) considerations: Determine if the patient needs assistive devices, such as hearing aids, eyeglasses, cane, walker, or dentures.

OPQRST METHOD OF HISTORY TAKING

O	Onset	The time that the symptoms associated with this event started.
P	Provocative; palliative. Positioning	That which makes it better; that which makes it worse. The position that the patient is in on arrival and the need to remain in this position or to move him or her.

Q	Quality of discomfort	Burning, stabbing, nagging, crushing, sharp, or dull.
R	Radiation of pain	Area to which the pain moves from the original site.
S	Severity of pain	Based on a 1-to-10 or other appropriate scale.
T	Time	Historical onset, such as earlier, similar events.

SAMPLE Method of History Taking

S	Signs and symptoms	Pain, bleeding, shortness of breath, injuries, fever, rash.
A	Allergies	Medications, environmental (foods, insects, plants, animals).
M	Medications	Prescribed, over-the-counter (OTC) vitamins/minerals, birth control and erectile dysfunction medications, herbal preparations, recreational drugs, other people's medications.
P	Past pertinent history	Especially related to the current event.
L	Last oral intake	Foods, fluids, other substances.
E	Events (precipitating)	Occurrence just prior to event.

Taking a History of Sensitive Topics

When asking a patient about **sensitive topics,** the AEMT should try to provide as much privacy as possible in an emergent situation in order to maintain confidentiality and protect the patient from reprisals. The AEMT should ask questions directly in a straightforward and nonjudgmental manner, stressing the need for information in order to help the patient, especially if the patient is reluctant to answer. Sensitive topics include the following:

- Sexual history: People who engage in unusual or unhealthy sexual practices, such as sadomasochism, autoerotic asphyxiation, swinging, and prostitution, are often reluctant to admit to those practices. Adolescents may be especially reluctant to admit they are pregnant or have engaged in sexual activity or have had an abortion. Males (especially those older than age 40) should be asked about the use of erectile dysfunction drugs (such as Viagra) because they are a contraindication to some medical treatments.
- Physical/Sexual abuse and/or violence: Victims often lie about abuse to defend the abuser or out of shame or fear of further violence.
- Alcohol/Drug use and abuse: Patients often underreport the extent of their drinking or drug taking or deny it altogether. Patients may be concerned about legal actions, such as if they have been driving drunk and gotten into an accident.

Special History-Taking Challenges

Special history-taking challenges include the following:

- Silent patient: Be patient, sensitive, and alert for nonverbal clues.
- Talkative patient: Allow the patient to speak freely for a few minutes and then periodically summarize.
- Anxious patient: Be patient, provide reassurance, and explain all procedures.
- Patient with multiple complaints: Ask the patient to help prioritize his or her issues.
- Hostile/angry patient: Remain calm; respond as appropriate.
- Intoxicated patient: Avoid cornering, belittling, or challenging the patient or asking the patient to lower his or her voice or stop swearing. Remain calm and treat the patient with respect.
- Depressed, crying patient: Question the severity of the patient's depression; listen and remain supportive and nonjudgmental.
- Patient with a language barrier: Use a translator if possible. Use hand gestures. Show the equipment before using it; point to the part of the body where the equipment will be used.

- Patient with a visual impairment: Announce your presence and explain all procedures verbally. Tell the patient before touching him or her.
- Patient with a hearing impairment: Determine if the patient has a hearing aid, and obtain it if possible. Speak slowly and clearly, facing the patient for any hearing deficit. If the patient has no hearing, use writing, hand gestures, and demonstrations to communicate.

SECONDARY ASSESSMENT

Following completion of the primary assessment and after attending to any life-threatening problems that are identified, carry out **a secondary assessment** as follows:

- Measure vital signs: Pulse (radial to carotid for adults and brachial for infants and small children), respiration rate, and BP. Using the correct BP cuff size is essential for accuracy. The length of the bladder in the cuff should be equal to 80% of the arm's circumference, and the lower edge of the cuff when positioned should end about one inch above the antecubital fossa (inner elbow). Inflate the cuff to 160 to 180 initially, and increase the pressure if pulse sounds are heard at that level.
- Ask further questions as indicated: This may focus on the primary complaint or others, depending on the situation.
- Conduct a physical examination: Examine the body; palpate for areas of tenderness or swelling; auscultate heart, lung, and abdominal sounds; and note any injuries. Do a brief head-to-toe assessment, and compare one side of the body with the other, noting any asymmetry.
- Treat any life-threatening injuries or conditions noted immediately.

ASSESSING THE PATIENT'S LEVEL OF CONSCIOUSNESS

The AVPU is a quick assessment done to determine the patient's level of consciousness. This may be one of the first assessments done when initially attending to a patient.

Alert, voice, pain, unresponsive (AVPU)			
A	Alert and awake; aware of person, place, time, and condition. Follows commands. Pediatric: Active and responds to external stimuli and to caregiver.	Yes	No
V	Responds to verbal stimuli, but the eyes do not open spontaneously. Pediatric: Responds only when the caregiver calls the child's name.	Yes	No
P	Responds to painful stimuli, such as pinching the skin/earlobe, but not to verbal stimuli. Pediatric: Responds only to painful stimuli, such as pinching the nailbed.	Yes	No
U	Unresponsive; does not respond to painful or verbal stimuli. Pediatric: Unresponsive.	Yes	No

ASSESSMENT OF LUNG SOUNDS

The lungs should be auscultated for normal and abnormal breath sounds.

Vesicular	Normal low-pitched sound over lung bases and most lung fields.
Bronchovesicular	Medium-pitched sound heard over the main bronchi. Duration is the same in expiration and inspiration.
Bronchial	Normal high-pitched loud sound heard over the trachea. The expiratory sound is as long or longer than the inspiratory sound. It is abnormal if it is heard over the lung bases.
Rales (crackles)	High-pitched crackles usually heard at the end of expiration in the lung bases, indicating fluid in the alveoli. May be fine or coarse.

Rhonchi	Deep rumbling sound may be high-pitched and sibilant (whistling) or low-pitched and sonorous (snoring) caused by constricted airways or large amounts of secretions in the airways. It is more pronounced on expiration.
Wheezes	High- or low-pitched whistling or musical sounds most pronounced on expiration. They often indicate asthma or a foreign-body obstruction.
Stridor	Crowing sound caused by inflammation and swelling of the larynx and trachea. Common finding in croup (associated with cough).
Grunts	Indicates respiratory distress in a newborn.
Friction rub	Grating sound heard over the area of the lungs where the pleura are inflamed.

BLOOD GLUCOSE MONITORING

Blood glucose monitoring is done with a glucometer. Testing is indicated with a decreased level of consciousness or confusion in a diabetic patient or decreased level of consciousness with the cause being unknown. The glucometer must be calibrated and tested regularly. Test results from capillary blood tend to be lower than test results on venous blood. The testing procedure includes the following:

- Wipe the site with an alcohol swab. The alcohol must be thoroughly dried before puncture, or it may interfere with the test results.
- Prick the side of the finger pad with a lancet or lancing device rather than the fingertip because the fingertip is more sensitive.
- Express a drop of blood onto the test strip.
- Insert the test strip into the glucometer according to the manufacturer's recommendations.
- Read the test results.
- Dispose of the lancet in a sharps container.

Warming the hand or lowering it may help to ensure adequate blood for the text. Hypoglycemia (low blood sugar/insulin reaction) is a reading at or below 70 mg/dL. Hyperglycemia (high blood sugar) is a reading at or above 160 mg/dL.

REASSESSMENT

Reassessment involves ongoing monitoring of the patient at regular intervals to determine changes in his or her condition or trends such as decreasing BP or increasing agitation. Reassessment is done after a secondary assessment. Unstable patients should be reassessed at least every 5 minutes and stable patients every 15 minutes. Reassessment should include reviewing the primary assessment, taking vital signs, repeating the physical examination (including evaluation of mental status), and monitoring the chief complaint and response to interventions. Reassessment findings should be compared to baseline findings. The patient's airway, ventilation, and circulation should be reassessed as well as the patient's degree of pain—stable, better, or worse. Each intervention should be reassessed for effectiveness and the need for modifications of treatment or if new interventions should be determined. If the patient is receiving oxygen, the tank and all of the equipment should be checked to ensure that they are functioning properly.

Medicine

ALTERED MENTAL STATUS

Altered mental status occurs because brain functioning is disrupted. Signs of altered mental status may be subtle (such as slight agitation, lethargy, sleepiness, or forgetfulness) or more obvious (such as disorientation, confusion, personality changes, violent behavior, somnolence, seizures, and coma). An altered mental status may occur abruptly or may have a slower onset, depending on the cause.

- Inadequate oxygenation: Brain cells can only survive about 6 minutes without oxygen, but damage begins to occur after about 60 seconds.
- Inadequate ventilation: Even if oxygen is plentiful, gas exchange is inadequate with impaired ventilation.
- Overdose of medication: May occur with numerous drugs, including opioids/narcotics (such as heroin and oxycodone), antipsychotics, hallucinogens, inhalants, cocaine, methamphetamines, and benzodiazepines.
- Poisoning: Includes arsenic; lead; cyanide; and overdose of medications such as acetaminophen, clonidine, salicylates, calcium channel blockers, and beta blockers.
- Infection: Systemic infections (sepsis), brain abscesses, chronic infections (human immunodeficiency virus/acquired immune deficiency syndrome [HIV/AIDS]).
- Psychological/psychiatric condition: Includes bipolar disorder, schizophrenia, post-traumatic stress disorder (PTSD), and depression.
- Diabetes: Hyperglycemia and hypoglycemia (especially insulin reaction).

NEUROLOGICAL SYSTEM

The **neurological (nervous) system** consists of the central nervous system ([CNS] brain, spinal cord and nerves) and the peripheral nervous system ([PNS] sensory neurons, ganglia [nerve clusters], and nerves connecting to the CNS). The brain consists of the cerebrum (frontal, temporal, parietal, and occipital lobes); the cerebellum; and the brain stem, which is continuous with the spinal cord. The PNS is divided into the autonomic nervous system (ANS) and the somatic nervous system (SoNS). The autonomic nervous system controls the body's organs and maintains homeostasis (balance). Functions of the ANS include control of the heart rate and function, respiration, digestion, sexual arousal, and other systems. The SoNS comprises cranial and spinal nerves that connect the CNS to the skeletal muscles and skin. The SoNS is the voluntarily controlled component of the PNS, and it receives and responds to external sensory stimuli from the skin and sensory organs.

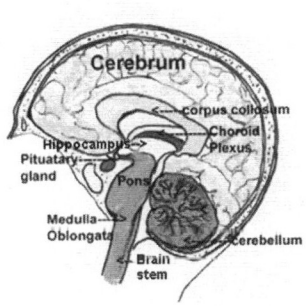

> **Review Video: Brain Anatomy**
> Visit mometrix.com/academy and enter code: 222476
>
> **Review Video: Somatic Nervous System**
> Visit mometrix.com/academy and enter code: 100382

ISCHEMIC AND HEMORRHAGIC STROKES

Strokes result from interruption of blood flow to an area of the brain. Ischemic strokes (80%) are caused by blockage of an artery supplying the brain, usually from a thrombus (blood clot) or embolus (traveling clot). Hemorrhagic strokes (20%) result from a ruptured cerebral artery, causing not only a lack of oxygen and nutrients but also edema (swelling) that causes widespread pressure and damage. With both types, patients may experience weakness, paralysis, and loss of sensation in one or more extremities; difficulty speaking or loss of speech; vision impairment; difficulty swallowing; headache; an altered state of consciousness (confusion, disorientation); or coma. Transient ischemic attacks (TIAs) from small clots cause similar but short-lived (minutes to hours) symptoms. Emergent treatment includes placing the patient in the semi-Fowlers or Fowler's position and administering oxygen. The patient may require oral suctioning if the secretions pool. The patient's airway, breathing, and circulation should be assessed. Patients should be transported immediately to the receiving facility because thrombolytic therapy to dissolve blood clots should be administered within 1 to 3 hours.

> **Review Video: Overview of Strokes**
> Visit mometrix.com/academy and enter code: 310572

CINCINNATI PREHOSPITAL STROKE SCALE

The Cincinnati Prehospital Stroke Scale should be administered to any patient who is suspected of having a stroke. The patient may be experiencing a stroke if testing positive for any of the three signs and should be transported to the receiving facility as soon as possible.

Signs	Directions to patient	Abnormal results
Facial drooping	Smile. Show your teeth.	One side of the face is weak or paralyzed and doesn't move as well as the other.
Arm drifting	Close your eyes and hold your arms out straight and hold them there for 10 seconds.	One arm doesn't move at all or drifts downward.
Speaking abnormality	Repeat after me: "Don't count your chickens before they are hatched."	Patient slurs words, uses inappropriate words, or is unable to respond.

LOS ANGELES PREHOSPITAL STROKE SCREEN

The **Los Angeles Prehospital Stroke Screen** is used to assess patients in a prehospital setting who have symptoms that suggest a stroke (such as altered state of consciousness, difficulty speaking, one-sided weakness, or paralysis). The results are positive for stroke if all criteria are met or are unable to be measured and the physical exam shows an unequal response. Note: A patient may still be having a stroke even if all the criteria are not met.

General criteria	Yes	No	Unknown
Age >45	X		
No history of epilepsy or seizures	X		
Onset of symptoms <24 hours	X		
Patient was able to walk before the onset of symptoms	X		
Blood glucose between 60 and 400 mg/dL	X		

Physical criteria	Equal	Right	Left
Facial smile	Normal	Droop	Droop
Grip strength	Normal	Weak or no grip	Weak or no grip
Arm strength	Normal	Drifts or falls down	Drifts or falls down

TYPES OF HEADACHES

Type of headache	Characteristics	Prehospital
Tension	Steady, constant pressure-like pain usually starting in the forehead, temples, or the back of the neck.	May vary depending on the cause and severity. Manage the patient's airway/ventilation/oxygen supplementation as needed, dim the lights, and place the patient in a position of comfort (usually semi-Fowler's or Fowler's), and apply a cold compress.
Cluster	Unilateral, occurring one to eight times daily, often for several weeks and associated with severe pain in the eye and orbit and radiating to the face and temporal area.	
Migraine	Severe recurring headaches often characterized by a prodrome phase, aura phase, headache phase, and recovery phase.	
Head/Neck trauma related	Vary but may start at neck or shoulders and radiate to the top of the head.	
Bleeding/Stroke related	<u>Epidural:</u> Sudden severe, intense. <u>Subdural:</u> Progressive headache worsening over time. <u>Subarachnoid:</u> "Thunderclap" severe headache with abrupt onset; it may be worse at the back of the head. <u>Stroke:</u> Tension-type headache with the site of pain relating to the area of injury. Often associated with alterations in mental status and other symptoms, such as weakness, paralysis, nausea and vomiting, and photophobia.	

SEIZURES

Seizures are sudden, involuntary, abnormal electrical disturbances in the brain that can manifest as alterations of consciousness, spastic tonic and clonic movements, convulsions, and loss of consciousness.

- Tonic-clonic (grand mal): Occurs without warning.
- Tonic period (10–30 seconds): The eyes roll upward with loss of consciousness, the arms flex, and the body stiffens in symmetric contractions with cyanosis and salivating.
- Clonic period (usually 30 seconds or longer): Violent rhythmic jerking with contraction and relaxation and sometimes incontinence of urine and feces.

During the seizure, the patient's head and body should be protected from injury but no attempt should be made to insert anything into the mouth or restrain the patient. If possible, the patient should be screened from spectators and turned onto his or her side (the recovery position) to prevent aspiration. Following seizures, there may be confusion, disorientation, and impairment of motor activity and speech and vision for several hours. Headache, nausea, and vomiting may occur. Prehospital: Monitor the airway, breathing, and circulation and suction and administer oxygen as needed. Insert a nasopharyngeal airway for assisted ventilation if the patient is cyanotic.

PARTIAL SEIZURES

Partial seizures are caused by an electrical discharge to a localized area of the cerebral cortex, such as the frontal, temporal, or parietal lobes with seizure characteristics related to the area of involvement. They may begin in a focal area and become generalized, often preceded by an aura.

- Simple partial: Unilateral motor symptoms including somatosensory, psychic, and autonomic.
- Aversive: Eyes and head are turned away from the focal side.
- Sylvan (usually during sleep): Tonic-clonic movements of the face, salivation, and arrested speech.
- Special sensory: Various sensations (numbness, tingling, prickling, or pain) spreading from one area. May include visual sensations, posturing, or hypertonia. These are rare in patients <8 years old.
- Complex (psychomotor): There is no loss of consciousness, but there may be altered levels of consciousness, and patients may be nonresponsive with amnesia. May involve complex sensorium with bad tastes, auditory or visual hallucinations, and a feeling of déjà vu or strong fear. Patients may carry out repetitive activities, such as walking, running, smacking lips, chewing, or drawling. Patients are rarely aggressive. The seizure is usually followed by prolonged drowsiness and confusion. Occurs from age 3 through adolescence.

Prehospital: Provide supportive care.

STATUS EPILEPTICUS

Status epilepticus (SE) is usually generalized tonic-clonic seizures that are characterized by a series of seizures with the intervening time being too short for the regaining of consciousness. The constant seizures and periods of apnea can lead to exhaustion, respiratory failure with hypoxemia and hypercapnia, hyperthermia, cardiac failure, and death. SE may result from uncontrolled epilepsy, noncompliance with anticonvulsive treatment, stroke, encephalopathy, drug toxicity, brain trauma, brain tumors (neoplasms), and metabolic disorders. SE is life threatening, so treatment should begin as soon as possible.

Prehospital care includes the following:

- Place an intravenous (IV) line.
- If opioid drug intoxication is the suspected cause, administer naloxone.
- Administer midazolam (intramuscular [IM]) (5 to 10 mg), lorazepam (IV), or diazepam (IV) to control seizures.
- Intubate and ventilate if in respiratory distress.
- Provide supportive care for seizures to prevent injury.
- Control hyperthermia with room-temperature water to skin and an IV normal saline (NS) bolus of 500 mL.

GLASGOW COMA SCALE (GCS)

The **Glasgow Coma Scale (GCS)** measures the depth and duration of coma or impaired levels of consciousness; it is used for postoperative assessment. The GCS measures three parameters: best eye response, best verbal response, and best motor response, with a total possible score that ranges from 3 to 15. The same scale is used with slight modifications for infants.

Eye opening	4: Spontaneous. 3: To verbal stimuli. 2: To pain (not of face). 1: No response.

Verbal	5: Oriented (Infant: Smiles, exhibits appropriate interactions). 4: Conversation is confused, but he or she can answer questions (Infant: Crying but consolable). 3: Uses inappropriate words (Infant: Moaning, sometimes inconsolable). 2: Speech incomprehensible (Infant: Inconsolable, agitated). 1: No response.
Motor	6: Moves on command (Infant: Moves spontaneously or with purpose). 5: Moves purposefully to respond to pain. 4: Withdraws in response to pain. 3: Decorticate posturing (flexion) in response to pain. 2: Decerebrate posturing (extension) in response to pain. 1: No response.

Injuries/conditions are classified according to the total score as follows: 3–8, coma; ≤ 8, severe head injury; 9–12, moderate head injury; 13–15, mild head injury.

ACUTE ABDOMEN

Acute abdomen is an acute intra-abdominal disorder that occurs with abrupt onset and usually requires emergency surgical intervention, although some patients may respond to other treatments, such as antibiotics. Acute abdomen may result from infection (peritonitis, pancreatitis, cholecystitis, appendicitis, diverticulitis), perforation, rupture of an internal organ (such as the spleen), aortic aneurysm, obstruction, infarction (necrotic tissue resulting from a blood clot or obstructed blood supply). If the blood supply is interrupted, gangrene may occur within 6 hours. Acute abdomen is characterized by inflammation, distension (often including guarding and rigidity), and acute pain (moderate/severe of fewer than 7 days' duration). Abdominal pain is especially concerning in pediatric and geriatric patients and those with impaired immune systems (such as HIV/AIDS patients and those receiving chemotherapy). Acute abdomen in infants and children may indicate conditions not commonly found in adults such as pyloric stenosis, volvulus, and necrotizing enterocolitis. Prehospital: Obtain a medical history regarding the quality, location, and duration of pain as well as referred pain; place the patient in a comfortable position; administer oxygen; and provide rapid transport.

GASTROINTESTINAL (GI) TRACT

Body part	Function
Mouth	Chews, moistens, begins carbohydrate hydrolysis (the breakdown of food by enzymes), creates a bolus of food. Connected to the esophagus by the pharynx.
Esophagus	Transports a bolus through the lower esophageal sphincter (which prevents backflow up the esophagus) to the stomach by peristalsis (wavelike contractions).
Stomach	Churns, secretes acids and enzymes, begins hydrolysis of proteins, and creates chyme (a more fluid substance).
Small intestine (about 20 feet long)	Duodenum: Accepts chyme and digests food to prepare for absorption. Jejunum: Absorbs most of the nutrients from the food, including vitamin B_{12}. Accepts bile from the liver and gallbladder to digest fats and pancreatic enzymes from the pancreas to digest proteins, fats, and carbohydrates. Ileum: Contains the ileocecal valve, which controls the flow of chyme into the large intestine.
Large intestine (about 5 feet long)	Cecum: Reabsorbs fluids and electrolytes. Appendix: Serves no function. Ascending, transverse, descending colon: Reabsorbs water, vitamin K, and electrolytes to form feces.
Rectum	Stores feces.

Body part	Function
Anus	Contains sphincters that control the expelling of feces.

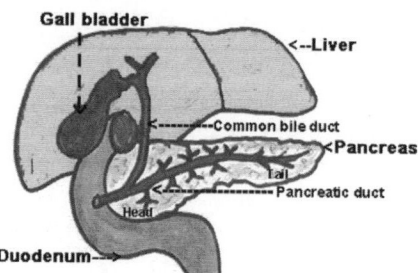

GASTROINTESTINAL (GI) BLEEDING

Upper **GI bleeding** (mouth to stomach) is characterized by nausea and hematemesis (vomiting of bright-red blood or partially digested, dark-brown, granulated ["coffee ground"] blood) and/or abdominal pain on palpation. With lower GI bleeding (small intestine to anus), the abdomen may be distended and tender and the patient may be passing blood through the anus. If bleeding has been slow and chronic, the patient may have only vague complaints of weakness and abdominal discomfort. In all cases, blood will mix with the stool. Melena (black-colored stool) usually indicates an upper GI bleed because the blood has been partially digested. Hematochezia (wine-colored stool or bright-red blood in the stool) indicates a lower GI bleed. Patients develop shock if blood loss is profound (≥40%). Prehospital: Examine the abdomen and note pain, monitor vital signs, and note signs of acute blood loss (fall in BP; increase in pulse; pallor; or cold, clammy skin). Provide suctioning if needed. Provide supplemental oxygen and ventilation as needed. Place the patient in the recovery position if he or she is vomiting. Place the patient flat with the feet elevated for shock.

ULCERATIVE COLITIS AND CROHN'S DISEASE

Ulcerative colitis is superficial inflammation of the mucosa of the colon and rectum, causing ulcerations ranging from pinpoint to extensive. Ulcerations may bleed and produce purulent material. The mucosa of the bowel becomes swollen, erythematous (red), and granular. Onset is usually between ages 15 and 30. Ulcerative colitis may affect only the rectum, the entire colon, or only the left colon. Indications include abdominal pain (usually absent or mild unless disease is severe), bloody diarrhea, rectal bleeding, fecal urgency, and tenesmus (a constant feeling of having to defecate). **Crohn's disease** is chronic inflammation of any area of the GI system but most commonly the small intestine and the beginning of the large intestine, resulting in ulcers that may involve the full thickness of the intestinal wall. An acute flare-up may mimic appendicitis. Indications include diarrhea (watery), rectal bleeding, abdominal cramping and pain (usually in the right lower quadrant), nausea, vomiting, fever, and night sweats. Prehospital: Provide supportive care, manage the patient's airway/ventilation/oxygen supplementation (to maintain oxygen saturation of ≥94%), and provide shock treatment per protocol if necessary.

PERITONITIS

Peritonitis is a bacterial infection of the peritoneum (lining of the abdominal cavity) that can lead to septicemia and death. Patients with kidney failure (especially those patients on peritoneal dialysis), liver disease, or infection of the GI tract are especially at risk. Other causes include an abdominal wound, ruptured appendix, perforated colon, diverticulitis, abdominal surgery, and inflammatory bowel disease. Symptoms include signs of acute abdomen: abdominal pain and distension, rigid abdomen, nausea and vomiting, diarrhea, fever, and chills. Other symptoms may include decreased urine output, excessive thirst, and tachycardia (rapid pulse). Peritonitis may be associated with ulcerative diseases, such as Crohn's disease (open sores through all layers of the walls of any part of the GI tract, most commonly in the ileum) and ulcerative colitis (open sores in the inner lining of the colon). Prehospital: Obtain an accurate medical history, note the condition of the abdomen with gentle palpation, provide supplemental oxygen/ventilation as needed, and position the patient for comfort because he or she may be experiencing severe pain.

Pediatric and Geriatric Patients with Abdominal Pain

Because **pediatric patients** (infants and small children) have large organs in relation to their size and very little protection with muscles or bone, organs such as the bladder, liver, and kidneys are more likely to suffer injury from abdominal trauma than they are in adults. Children have smaller rib cages and pelvic bones, so the abdomen is more vulnerable. Abdominal pain in children may be associated with constipation (right lower quadrant pain) as well as appendicitis, which is characterized by right lower quadrant pain and a lack of appetite, but it may be hard to identify in children because they may not have appreciable or localized pain initially. Pain persisting for ≥48 hours usually indicates rupture of the appendix. Vomiting and diarrhea may rapidly deplete fluids because of lower fluid volume, resulting in dehydration. **Geriatric patients** with acute abdomen may not exhibit typical abdominal rigidity or guarding. Additionally, abdominal pain may be an indication of a heart attack rather than a GI problem.

Allergic Reactions and Anaphylaxis

Allergic reactions are a response of the body's immune system to an antigen (substance), such as peanuts or shellfish. The body produces antibodies (immunoglobulins, such as IgE or non-IgE) that can identify and try to neutralize or destroy antigens. Allergic responses may be mild (local rash, redness, itching, swelling, congestion), moderate (generalized itching, difficulty breathing), or severe (life-threatening anaphylaxis). With **anaphylaxis**, an antigen triggers the release of substances that affect the skin, cardiopulmonary system, and GI system. Histamine causes initial redness and swelling by inducing vasodilation. In some cases, initial reactions may be mild, but subsequent contact can cause severe life-threatening response. Symptoms include the following: a sudden onset of weakness, dizziness, and confusion; tachycardia; generalized swelling; itching; severe low BP leading to shock; airway obstruction; nausea and vomiting; hives; diarrhea; seizures; coma; and death. Prehospital: For hypotension and facial swelling, respiratory distress, or swelling of the mouth, provide epinephrine (if authorized) or assist with an autoinjector to the lateral thigh and repeat every 5–10 minutes as needed, provide supplemental oxygen/ventilation, and transport immediately.

Infectious and Contagious Diseases

Infectious diseases, which may be communicable or noncommunicable, are those that are caused when microorganisms (such as bacteria, viruses, retroviruses, protozoa, helminths [worms] and fungi) invade the body and cause disease. Noncommunicable diseases may spread from an environmental source, such as contaminated water or food (such as with food poisoning), or from insects that carry the disease (such as with Lyme disease). However, they do not spread from person to person, so only standard precautions are needed when caring for these patients. Contagious diseases are infections that are communicable from person to person. They may be spread through direct physical contact and sneezing or coughing as well as through contact with blood or other body fluids (feces, semen, urine, or perspiration). With contagious diseases, the type of precautions needed depends on the mode of infection and they may range from contact to droplet to airborne precautions; the type of PPE needed also varies.

Decontaminating an Ambulance

Decontaminating an ambulance begins with removal of any debris, with sharps being deposited in a sharps container and soiled linen being red-bagged. Then, the equipment and surfaces that have had contact with a patient or with contaminated materials must be cleaned, disinfected, or sterilized, depending on the type of equipment/surface and the type of contamination. Between patients, surfaces and equipment should be wiped down with a disinfectant, such as a 1:100 bleach solution or premixed wipes. Alcohol-based products are effective for many organisms, but not for *Clostridioides difficile* (which is spread through fecal contamination). If equipment is left with a patient at a receiving facility, that facility must clean the equipment or place it in a red bag before returning it. At the end of the day, the entire ambulance should be cleaned. Various methods of sterilization, including the use of a fogging agent and UV lights, are available. All cleaning procedures must be recorded for compliance purposes.

HUMAN IMMUNODEFICIENCY VIRUS/ACQUIRED IMMUNE DEFICIENCY SYNDROME

Human immunodeficiency virus infection (HIV) is the retrovirus that causes **acquired immune deficiency syndrome (AIDS)**. Diagnosis is determined by the CD4+ T-cell count with AIDS currently being diagnosed with a CD4+ count of <200 cells per mm^3. HIV is transmitted in bodily fluids (blood, semen, vaginal secretions, and breast milk) that contain free virions and infected CD4+ T-cells. The categories are as follows:

- Category A (CD4+ count <500): Asymptomatic or lymphadenopathy, sore throat, and fatigue.
- Category B (CD4+ count 200 to 499): Conditions include candidiasis, pelvic inflammatory disease, bacillary angiomatosis, fever, diarrhea, herpes zoster, low platelet count, weight loss, and peripheral neuropathy.
- Category C (AIDS) (CD4+ count <200): Invasive diseases are common. Conditions include cervical cancer, candidiasis, cytomegalovirus, encephalopathy, TB, *Pneumocystis jirovecii* pneumonia (formerly known as *P. carinii* pneumonia), Kaposi's sarcoma, toxoplasmosis, and wasting syndrome.

About 1.2 million people in the United States have HIV infection, but 13% are unaware of it. Risk factors include unprotected sex, especially males having sex with other males, and needle sharing. Prehospital: Provide supportive care, manage the airway, support ventilation, and provide IV access if necessary. Use droplet precautions for cough.

HEPATITIS AND FULMINANT HEPATITIS

Hepatitis, inflammation of the liver, is caused by bacteria, viruses, or exposure to toxic chemicals, including alcohol or drugs. However, viral infection is most common and may be foodborne or bloodborne, although only bloodborne diseases, hepatitis B and C, cause chronic liver disease. Symptoms include jaundice (yellowing of the skin, eyes) and clay-colored stool from impaired excretion of bile, dark urine, abdominal pain, flu-like symptoms, nausea and vomiting, loss of appetite, itching, and increased risk of bleeding.

Fulminant hepatitis is an acute inflammation of the liver that may be caused by viruses, toxic substances, or overdose with acetaminophen and can result in encephalopathy, liver failure, and death within 1 to 72 days. Vaccinations are available for hepatitis A virus (HAV) and hepatitis B virus (HBV). Treatment for accidental exposure to HAV is prophylaxis with HAV immune globulin, and that for HBV is initiating vaccinations if the patient is unvaccinated or HBV immune globulin. Prehospital: Use standard precautions, provide supportive care as needed, manage the patient's airway/ventilation, and provide IV fluids if necessary.

HEPATITIS INFECTIONS AND MODES OF TRANSMISSION

Type of hepatitis	Transmission	Characteristics
Hepatitis A (HAV)	Foodborne/oral-fecal, oral-anal sex	Usually mild infection (may be asymptomatic) lasting about 2 months.
Hepatitis B (HBV)	Bloodborne/blood and body fluids/sex, needle sharing	Most common bloodborne hepatitis and very infectious. Most recover within 6 months, but up to 10% develop chronic disease, which can lead to liver failure or liver cancer, and they become carriers.
Hepatitis C (HCV)	Bloodborne/blood and body fluids/sex/needle sharing	Causes chronic infection and is the most common cause of liver transplantation. May be asymptomatic for 20 years.
Hepatitis D (HDV)	Bloodborne/blood and body fluids/sex/needle sharing	Co-infection with HBV and increases the risk of developing fulminant hepatitis and cirrhosis.
Hepatitis E (HEV)	Foodborne/oral-fecal, oral-anal sex	Usually found in travelers from South Asia or Africa from areas with poor sanitation. It is a mild form similar to HAV.

Type of hepatitis	Transmission	Characteristics
Hepatitis G (HGV-C)	Bloodborne/blood and body fluids/sex/needle sharing	Believed to be a variation of type C and can be a co-infection of HBV and HBC. Usually a mild infection, but it may be chronic.

ENDOCRINE SYSTEM AND HORMONES PRODUCED

Hypothalamus	Links the endocrine and nervous systems. Produces hormones that are stored in the posterior lobe of the pituitary gland, and stimulates the pituitary to release hormones.
Pineal gland	Secretes melatonin and dimethyltryptamine, which control sleep cycles and dreaming.
Pituitary gland	The posterior lobe secretes oxytocin (it stimulates uterine contractions/lactation) and vasopressin (aka antidiuretic hormone) (it raises BP and promotes water reabsorption). The anterior lobe secretes hormones that control cell growth (somatotropin), body growth (growth hormone), release of hormones by the thyroid (thyrotropin), release of steroids from the adrenal glands (corticotropin), and reproductive functions (follicle-stimulating hormone and luteinizing hormone).
Thyroid gland	Secretes hormones that control protein production, basal metabolic rate, and oxygen consumption (T3, T4, and calcitonin).
Parathyroid glands	Secretes parathyroid hormone, which controls the use of calcium.
Adrenal glands	Produce cortisol (roles in metabolism), aldosterone (water and sodium levels), and androgens (male hormones).
Ovaries	Secrete female hormones (estrogen and progesterone).
Testes	Secrete androgens (testosterone).

> **Review Video: Endocrine System**
> Visit mometrix.com/academy and enter code: 678939

DIABETIC CONDITIONS

Diabetes mellitus is a group of metabolic disorders that involve hyperglycemia (increased blood glucose [sugar]) because of defective production and/or action of insulin. Insulin metabolizes glucose to produce energy as fuel for body cells.

- Type 1: Autoimmune destruction of beta cells in the pancreas results in no or deficient insulin production. Treatment: Insulin. Symptoms: Rapid onset, increased thirst, frequent urination, increased hunger, delayed healing, weight loss, frequent infections, and blurred vision.
- Type 2: Insulin baseline may be normal or deficient, but there is no or an inadequate increase in response to a meal, so the glucose level rises but there is decreased uptake by the tissues. Insulin resistance occurs because there is decreased sensitivity to insulin by the tissues. Type 2 diabetes is often related to obesity. Treatment is with oral diabetic agents. Symptoms include slow onset, increased thirst, increased urination, candidal (fungal) infections, delayed healing, and weight gain.
- Gestational: Beta cells in the pancreas are unable to produce adequate insulin during pregnancy, but normal production resumes after delivery. Treatment varies. Symptoms include being asymptomatic or having increased thirst and urinary frequency.

Pediatric patients with diabetes mellitus most commonly have type 1 and are insulin dependent with the peak age for onset happening during adolescence; however, rates of type 2 diabetes are increasing in young children and adolescents, especially if they are overweight. Children (especially <15) with late stages of hyperglycemia may develop cerebral edema with headache and weakness and changes in mental status, particularly irritability. Children are also more likely to develop hypoglycemia than are adults and are more prone to having seizures and becoming dehydrated than are adults. Hypoglycemia may result from excessive exercise. Many children may be undiagnosed and may present with diabetic ketoacidosis.

Geriatric patients often have reduced sensation because of neuropathy associated with diabetes, and they may be unaware of injuries. Geriatric patients are also prone to developing dehydration and infections. Diabetes is the leading cause of lower limb amputation and kidney failure, so many patients with amputations and on hemodialysis are diabetic. Patients with diabetes may have an atypical presentation of a myocardial infarction (heart attack) without chest pain.

Hyperglycemia

Hyperglycemia is high blood glucose (sugar) with a level of greater than 130mg/dL after fasting for 8 hours or greater than 180 mg/dL 2 hours after eating. Hyperglycemia may occur in undiagnosed diabetic patients or in diabetic patients who have taken inadequate insulin; those who have eaten a diet too high in carbohydrates (sugars); or those who are ill, such as with an infection. Initial signs include polyuria (increased urine), polyphagia (hunger), polydipsia (increased thirst), headaches, lethargy, fatigue, and blurred vision, but if blood sugar is very high (greater than 250 mg/dL), then patients may become increasingly somnolent, and the patient may develop diabetic ketoacidosis from the buildup of ketones as fat is broken down by the body for energy because sugar/glucose cannot be used. The patient may exhibit Kussmaul's breathing (fruity-smelling breath from ketones), could lapse into a coma, and could die if left untreated. Prehospital: Question the patient about diabetes and the use of diabetic medications. Check the patient's blood sugar level; monitor the vital signs and oxygen saturation, and provide supportive care as needed. Rapid transport is required with altered levels of consciousness.

Hyperglycemic Hyperosmolar Nonketotic Syndrome (HHNS) or Coma (HHNK)

Hyperglycemic hyperosmolar nonketotic syndrome (HHNS) or coma (HHNK) occurs in people without a history of diabetes or in people with mild type 2 diabetes but with insulin resistance resulting in persistent hyperglycemia, which causes osmotic diuresis. Fluid shifts from intracellular to extracellular spaces to maintain osmotic equilibrium, but the increased glycosuria and dehydration result in hypernatremia and increased osmolality (concentration). This condition is most common in persons 50–70 years old, and it often is precipitated by an acute illness such as a stroke, medications such as thiazides, or dialysis treatments. HHNS differs from ketoacidosis because although the insulin level is not adequate, it is high enough to prevent the breakdown of fat. Symptoms include polyuria, dehydration, hypotension, tachycardia, blood glucose >500 mg/dL, changes in mental status, hallucinations, seizures, and hemiparesis. Prehospital: Question the patient about his or her history of diabetes and use of diabetes medications. Check the patient's blood sugar level, monitor the vital signs and oxygen saturation, and provide supportive care as needed. Rapid transport is needed for altered levels of consciousness.

Hypoglycemia

Hypoglycemia (low blood sugar/glucose) is most often caused by an insulin reaction (too much insulin for the amount of glucose/sugar intake) or an overdose of oral diabetes medications, which stimulate the overproduction of insulin. Hypoglycemia may occur if patients took insulin but skipped a meal, vomited, or exercised too strenuously, depleting the body of sugar/glucose while insulin levels remain high. Increased insulin levels cause glucose levels to fall to at or below 70 mg/dL, initially resulting in tremors, headache, blurred vision dizziness, and pallor leading to confusion, bizarre behavior, lack of coordination, combative behavior, personality changes, tachycardia, and irregular heartbeat. Severe hypoglycemia may lead to seizures, coma, and death. Hypoglycemia is life threatening if untreated. Infants may have dehydration and seizures; geriatric patients may have dehydration and stroke. Prehospital: Ask the patient about his or her diabetes status and use of diabetes medications. Check the patient's glucose level, and administer oral glucose tablets, one tablespoon of sugar, or a glass of orange juice if the patient is able to swallow; provide rapid transport for altered levels of consciousness.

INSULIN

Insulin is used to metabolize glucose when the pancreas does not produce insulin in cases of type 1 diabetes mellitus. Patients may need to take a combination of insulins (short and long acting) to maintain glucose control. The duration of action may vary according to the individual's metabolism, intake, and level of activity:

- Rapid acting (lispro [Humalog], aspart [Novolog], glulisine [Apidra]): Onset within 10–30 minutes, peaks between 30–90 minutes, and lasts 3–5 hours.
- Short acting (regular [R] [Humulin, Novolin, or Velosulin for insulin pump]): Onset within 30–60 minutes, peaks in 2–5 hours, and lasts 5–8 hours. Velosulin has an onset in 30 to 60 minutes, peaks in 1–2 hours, and lasts 2–3 hours.
- Intermediate acting (NPH [N]): Onset in 1–2 hours, peaks at 4–12 hours, and lasts 16–24 hours.
- Long acting (insulin glargine [Lantus/Basaglar] and insulin detemir [Levemir]): Lantus and Basaglar—Onset in 1–1.5 hours, no peak time, and lasts 20–24 hours. Levemir—Onset in 1–2 hours, peaks in 6–8 hours, and lasts up to 24 hours.
- Ultralong acting (insulin degludec [Tresiba]): Onset in 30–90 minutes, no peak, and lasts 42 hours.
- Combined/Premixed (NPH/Regular [70/30 or 50/50 or various other combinations]): Onset in 15–30 minutes, peaks at 2–12 hours (depending on the combination), and lasts 16–24 hours.

ORAL HYPOGLYCEMIC AGENTS

Sulfonylureas **First generation: acetohexamide, chlorpropamide, tolazamide, and tolbutamide** **Second generation: glipizide, glyburide, glimepiride**	These increase the production of insulin by the pancreas. They are more effective early in treatment, but they become less effective over time.
Meglitinides **repaglinide,** **nateglinide**	These increase the production of insulin by the pancreas. They are faster acting than sulfonylureas. They are taken 30 minutes prior to a meal up to the time of the meal so that they increase insulin production during and after the meal.
Biguanides **metformin,** **metformin with glyburide**	These reduce glucose production by the liver. They are often taken as part of combination therapy with another drug.
Alpha-glucosidase inhibitors **acarbose**	These slow the absorption of carbohydrates by the intestines. They are not effective for people with fasting hyperglycemia.
Thiazolidinediones **pioglitazone, rosiglitazone**	These improve insulin sensitivity, transport, and utilization. They are most effective for people with insulin resistance, but they do not increase the production of insulin, although they may be combined with another drug. Rosiglitazone has restricted use because of the risk of heart attack.

ASSESSMENT OF PSYCHIATRIC PATIENTS

Assessment of patients with psychological/psychiatric symptoms should begin with a history that includes the patient's age and cultural/spiritual background and whether the patient has experienced similar symptoms previously or has a history of a psychiatric disorder as well as any history of substance abuse. Assessment includes the following:

- General appearance: Note hygiene, grooming, appropriate dress, eye contact, unusual movements (twitching, posturing, repetitive movements), and the appearance and condition of the skin.
- Speech: Note speech cadence and abnormal word use, such as neologisms (invented words), clang associations (rhyming), word salad (string of random words), and associative looseness (ideas shifting from one to another).

- Posture/Gait: Note automatisms (purposeless behaviors, such as drumming fingers), slowed motions, waxy flexibility (maintaining an awkward position for extended periods of time), ability to walk, and abnormalities of gait.
- Mental status: Note the patient's state of being alert versus nonalert, responsive versus nonresponsive, and coherent versus noncoherent; clarity of ideas; suicidal ideation; and desire for self-harm.
- Mood and affect: Note facial expressions, expressed emotions, and affect (blunted, broad, flat, inappropriate, restricted).
- Memory/Intellectual processes: Note if memory and intellectual processes are intact or impaired. Is the patient disoriented and confused or alert and responsive?
- Attention: Note if the patient's attention is focused or unfocused.

BEHAVIORAL ALTERATIONS

Behavioral alterations may include agitation, anger, throwing temper tantrums (children), acting aggressively (adolescents/adult), exhibiting poor judgment, and acting inappropriately. Behavioral alterations may result from psychiatric disorders (such as depression, schizophrenia, and bipolar disorder) and psychiatric medications as well as numerous other causes, including the following:

- Hypoglycemia/Low blood sugar (insulin reaction).
- Lack of adequate oxygen interferes with brain function.
- Shock (low BP; a rapid pulse results in inadequate blood supply to the brain).
- Mind-altering substances (cocaine, methamphetamine, lysergic acid diethylamide [LSD], Rohypnol [the date-rape drug]).
- Brain infection (meningitis, encephalitis, brain abscess).
- Seizure disorders (epilepsy, other causes of seizures).
- Poisoning/Overdose (lead poisoning, drug overdose).
- Malnutrition resulting in inadequate nourishment of brain tissue.
- Substance abuse (drug or alcohol abuse/withdrawal).
- Heat extremes (hypothermia/hyperthermia).

Indications of being a danger to self or others include severe agitation, hallucinations, delusional thinking, paranoia, self-destructive behavior (cutting, drug/alcohol abuse, promiscuity, risk-taking activities), depression, and suicide attempts. A patient may pose a risk to others if he or she is behaving in a threatening or violent manner and has a weapon (club, gun, knife, baseball bat).

CALMING PATIENTS WITH BEHAVIORAL EMERGENCIES

Patients with **behavioral emergencies** are often agitated and may be confused, fearful, and/or aggressive, so the AEMT must remain calm and approach the patient slowly; remain at a safe distance; and avoid fast movements, threatening postures, or attempts at physical contact, acknowledging the patient's agitation and offering assistance ("I can see that you're upset, and I want to help") and maintaining eye contact (unless the person is violent and reacts aggressively). The AEMT should encourage the patient to talk about what is causing the behavior and should answer questions honestly while avoiding threatening, arguing, or challenging the patient. If the patient is suffering hallucinations or delusional thinking, the AEMT should avoid playing along ("I don't see what you do") but should also avoid contradicting the patient directly when responding. Family or friends may assist with intervention. The AEMT should not leave the patient unattended and should try to lower distressing stimuli (such as lights and noise) and consider contacting law enforcement. Restraints should be avoided if possible.

SUICIDAL IDEATION

Suicidal ideation occurs frequently in those with mood disorders or depression (common in geriatric patients). Although females are more likely to attempt suicide, males actually successfully commit suicide three times more often than females, primarily because females tend to take overdoses from which they can be revived whereas males choose more violent means (jumping from a high place, shooting, or hanging). This holds true for adolescents and adults. Risk factors include psychiatric disorders (schizophrenia, bipolar disorder, post-traumatic stress disorder [PTSD], and substance abuse), physical disorders (HIV/AIDS, diabetes, traumatic brain injury, spinal cord injury), and social problems (bullying).

Passive suicidal ideation involves wishing to be dead or thinking about dying without making plans, whereas active suicidal ideation involves making plans. Patients at risk should be questioned about their feelings, problems, plans for suicide, and access to weapons. High-risk findings include the following:

- Violent suicide attempt (knives, gunshots) or access to a weapon.
- History of a suicide attempt and a suicide attempt with a low chance of rescue.
- Ongoing psychosis or disordered thinking.
- Ongoing severe depression and feelings of helplessness.
- Lack of a social support system.

AGITATED/EXCITED DELIRIUM

Patients with **agitated/excited delirium** are often very combative, aggressive, violent, and uncooperative, and they exhibit shouting, threaten violence, and behave bizarrely. The patient may experience hallucinations, disorientation, paranoia, and panic. Patients may be exceptionally strong and seem insensitive to pain. They are often hyperthermic (high temperature). Agitated/Excited delirium may be associated with hypoglycemia, brain damage, chemical imbalance, and substance abuse (methamphetamine, cocaine, phencyclidine [PCP], "angel dust"], and LSD). Patients often require restraints for their own or for others' safety, but they are at risk of death by asphyxiation or restraint (positional) because they fight desperately against the restraints. Prehospital: The AEMT should use active listening and try to establish rapport while assessing the patient's intellectual functioning, orientation, judgment and thought processes, language, mood, and appearance to determine if law enforcement or other assistance is needed. The patient may refuse care, but implied consent is legal for patients with abnormal behavior. The patient must be transported safely for treatment. The AEMT should look for medications or drugs on site and take them to the receiving facility.

RESTRAINTS

Patients needing restraints are often agitated, confused, and refuse care, but implied consent is legal for patients with abnormal behavior. **Restraints** include the following:

- Verbal: Try to calm the patient while being firm.
- Nonverbal: Use body language and a show of force (with a number of EMS personnel being present) to convince the patient.
- Physical: Use standard precautions; one person is assigned to each limb, while a fifth person reassures and tries to calm the patient. Apply multiple restraints as necessary, including across the trunk, being careful not to restrict the patient's breathing.
- Chemical: Use as a last resort (usually after physical restraints). Includes benzodiazepines (lorazepam) and neuroleptics (haloperidol).
- Tasers/Electrical stun guns: These may be used by law enforcement to subdue a severely agitated patient. They may cause burns, dart injuries, fall injuries, or cardiac arrest. Stun guns require direct contact, but Tasers may be shot from 20 feet away.

Document the reason for restraint, the types of restraints, the restraint technique, and the time the patient is restrained. Monitor the patient's condition continuously, including the heart rate, airway/ventilation/oxygen supplementation, and circulation.

CIRCULATORY SYSTEM

The **circulatory system** is responsible for the oxygenation of cells, perfusion (carrying of blood with oxygen, glucose, and nutrients to the cells), and gas exchange (removing waste products, such as carbon dioxide). The circulatory system serves as a blood reservoir (5 L), maintains blood pH (7.35–7.45) through a buffer system, responds to infections, and facilitates coagulation (blood clotting). The heart is located between the lungs and under and to the left of the mediastinum (breastbone). The heart has four chambers: upper (right atrium, left atrium) and lower (right ventricle and left ventricle). The myocardium (heart muscle) receives blood from two major coronary arteries and their branches. The inner lining of the heart is the endocardium, and the lining that surrounds the heart is the pericardium, which has an inner double-layered serous membrane (visceral pericardium) and a fibrous outer layer (parietal pericardium). The cardiac cycle involves one complete heartbeat with systole (ventricular contraction) and diastole (relaxation) phases. Stroke volume is the volume of blood ejected from the left ventricle in one cardiac cycle (about 60–70 mL), and cardiac output is the heart rate times the stroke volume.

The venous system includes the veins, venules, and venous capillaries, and it brings blood back to the heart via the inferior and superior vena cava. The arterial system includes the coronary arteries, which branch from the aorta after it leaves the heart; arteries; arterioles; and arterial capillaries. **The blood flows** as follows:

- Deoxygenated venous blood returns to the heart per the inferior vena cava, superior vena cava, and coronary sinus (bringing blood from the coronary arteries) into the right atrium, and then it flows through the tricuspid valve into the right ventricle.
- From the right ventricle, blood flows through the pulmonic (semilunar) valve into the pulmonary artery and to the lungs to exchange carbon dioxide for oxygen.
- Oxygenated blood flows from the lungs through the pulmonary veins into the left atrium and through the mitral (bicuspid) valve into the left ventricle.
- From the left ventricle, blood flows through the aortic valve and into the aorta, the coronary arteries, and the general circulation through the thoracic and abdominal aorta.

After blood flows through the valves, they close to prevent backflow. Both atria and both ventricles contract simultaneously.

COMPONENTS OF THE BLOOD

Blood cells are produced in the bone marrow. Blood is a viscous, dark-red fluid comprised of cells, gases, and plasma (55%). Blood components include the following:

- Erythrocytes (red blood cells [RBCs]): RBCs carry hemoglobin, which transports oxygen. If the RBC count is low (such as from blood loss) or the oxygen-carrying capacity is impaired (such as with anemia), the patient may experience hypoxemia (low oxygen). The life cycle of RBCs is normally 120 days.
- Leukocytes (white blood cells [WBCs]): WBCs defend the body against invading organisms (viruses, bacteria, fungi, and parasites), and in the bloodstream and tissues they respond to allergies. WBCs include lymphocytes (B, T, natural killer, and null cells), monocytes, eosinophils, basophils, and neutrophils.
- Thrombocytes (platelets): Platelets release clotting factors and have an active role in forming blood clots.
- Plasma (55% of blood): Plasma carries water, proteins, electrolytes, lipids (fats), blood cells, and glucose as well as clotting factors.

The primary blood types are A, B, AB, and O. Blood is either Rh– or RH+, and patients must receive transfusions of blood that are type and Rh compatible.

ANGINA AND HEART ATTACK

Chest pain may indicate angina (pain from temporary constriction/blockage of blood flow in the coronary arteries) or a heart attack (pain caused by blockage of blood flow to the heart muscle because of a blood clot [most common] or hemorrhage, resulting in the death of heart tissue). Heart problems in children are often associated with congenital heart disease. Geriatric and female patients may not have chest pain with a heart attack. Make note of the following:

- Character, location, and severity of the pain.
- Radiation of pain to the neck, jaw, arms, back, jaw, and/or stomach.
- Shortness of breath at rest or with exertion or worsening when lying flat.
- Skin: Cold, clammy skin is common with a heart attack.
- Vital signs: Note BP, pulse (rapid, irregular, slow), and respirations.
- Other: Note nausea and/or vomiting and dizziness/lightheadedness.

Prehospital: Provide the patient with a position of comfort (often semi-Fowler's if there is shortness of breath), provide a high concentration of oxygen with a nonrebreather mask, question the patient about medications taken recently and/or medications taken for pain (such as aspirin or nitroglycerin), and provide rapid transport.

Perfusion, Oxygenation of Tissues, and Cardiac Compromise

Perfusion depends on an adequate supply of red blood cells, which carry oxygen. Perfusion may be impaired if the heart does not pump adequately, if the rate of heart contractions is too low or too rapid to be effective, and if the volume of blood and/or red blood cells pumped is not adequate to provide oxygenation to the tissues. With adequate perfusion, **oxygenation of tissues** occurs when blood flows throughout the body, and gas exchange of carbon dioxide and waste products for oxygen occurs at the capillaries. **Cardiac compromise** results in inadequate circulation and/or perfusion of vital organs. Cardiac compromise may result from atherosclerosis (plaques/fatty deposits) in the arterial lumens, resulting in obstructed blood flow and inadequate dilation and constriction of arteries. Ischemia (low oxygenation) occurs with decreased blood flow and can damage tissues, but occlusion (obstruction) can result in the death of tissue. Cardiac compromise may result from heart damage causing an inadequate heart rate and/or pumping. Cardiac compromise may also result from an inadequate volume of circulating blood.

Management of a Patient with Chest Pain

Management of a patient with chest pain begins with a thorough assessment, primary and secondary survey, and use of the OPQRST and SAMPLE methods of history taking. Patients are often very frightened, so the AEMT should provide clear feedback and reassurance. The patient should be placed in the semi-Fowler's position, especially if he or she is experiencing shortness of breath, and the oxygen saturation should be monitored. Respiratory compromise may require supplemental oxygen, bag-mask ventilation (BVM) assistance, PEEP, CPAP/BiPAP, manually triggered ventilators (MTVs), or automatic transport ventilators (ATVs). The AEMT should determine the need for the assistance of an advanced emergency medical technician (AEMT) or a paramedic.

Pharmacological interventions (assist the patient with medication administration, or administer the medication according to protocol) may include the following:

- Aspirin (for suspected heart attack; Bayer, Heartline, ZORprin, Empirin): Provide 162 to 325 mg chewable (preferred). Contraindicated with GI bleeding, stroke.
- Nitroglycerin (for suspected angina; Nitro-Dur, Nitrolingual, NitroMist): Provide 0.4 mg sublingually repeated every 3–5 minutes up to three doses. Contraindicated if the patient has recently taken Viagra, had a stroke, or has excessive bleeding.
- Oral glucose (for suspected hypoglycemia/insulin reaction): Glucose tablets, solution.

All patients with chest pain should be transported because even mild chest discomfort may indicate that the patient is having a heart attack, especially in older patients and female patients, who often have atypical symptoms.

Cardiogenic Shock

Cardiogenic shock in adults is usually secondary to myocardial infarction damage of >40% of the left ventricle, reducing contractibility, interfering with the pumping mechanism of the heart, and decreasing oxygen perfusion. Characteristics include increased preload, increased afterload, and decreased contractibility. Together, these result in decreased cardiac output and an increase in systemic vascular resistance (SVR) to compensate and protect the vital organs. As the cardiac output decreases, tissue perfusion decreases, coronary artery perfusion decreases, fluid backs up, and the left ventricle fails to adequately pump the blood, resulting in pulmonary edema and right ventricular failure. Indications: Hypotension with systolic BP <90 mm Hg; tachycardia >100 beat/min with weak, thready pulse and dysrhythmias; decreased heart sounds; chest pain; tachypnea and basilar rales; pallor; and cool, moist skin. Prehospital: Manage the patient's airway/ventilation/oxygenation/intubation as needed; install an IV access line with fluid resuscitation; monitor the electrocardiogram (ECG), vital signs, and cardiac status; and provide inotropic/vasopressor (norepinephrine, dopamine) support.

Hypertensive Crisis

Hypertensive crisis (aka malignant hypertension) is a marked elevation in BP that can cause severe organ damage if left untreated. Causes include encephalopathy, intracranial hemorrhage, aortic dissection, eclampsia, and heart failure. Classifications are as follows:

- **Hypertensive emergency**: Acute hypertension, usually >120 mm Hg diastolic; it must be treated immediately to lower the BP in order to prevent damage to vital organs, such as the heart, brain, or kidneys.
- **Hypertensive urgency**: Acute hypertension must be treated within a few hours, but the vital organs are not in immediate danger. The blood pressure is lowered more slowly to avoid hypotension, ischemia of vital organs, or failure of autoregulation with a one-third reduction in 6 hours.

Symptoms include headache, dizziness, dyspnea, weakness, visual disturbances, anxiety, chest pain (atypical), heart failure, acute coronary syndrome, and stroke. Prehospital: Asymptomatic hypertension requires referral to a physician, whereas severe symptoms require rapid transport. Interventions include airway support/ventilation with oxygen supplementation and advanced life support as needed. Patients with severe dyspnea and pulmonary edema may need CPAP.

Angina Pectoris (Stable)

Impairment of blood flow through the coronary arteries leads to ischemia of the cardiac muscle and **angina pectoris**—pain that may occur in the sternum, chest, neck, arms (especially the left arm), or back. The pain frequently occurs with crushing pain substernally, radiating down the left arm or both arms, although this type of pain is more common in males than females, whose symptoms may appear less acute and may include nausea, shortness of breath, and fatigue. Elderly or diabetic patients may also have pain in their arms, no pain at all (silent ischemia), or weakness and numbness in both arms. Stable angina episodes usually last for <5 minutes and are fairly predictable exercise-induced episodes caused by atherosclerotic lesions blocking >75% of the lumen of the affected coronary artery. Precipitating events include exercise; a decrease in the environmental temperature; heavy eating; strong emotions (such as fright or anger); or exertion, including coitus. Stable angina episodes usually resolve in less than 5 minutes by decreasing the activity level and administering sublingual nitroglycerin. Provide supportive care, oxygen, and assist the patient to take nitroglycerin if available.

Angina Pectoris (Unstable, Variant/Prinzmetal's)

Unstable angina (also known as preinfarction or crescendo angina) is a progression of coronary artery disease, and it occurs when there is a change in the pattern of stable angina. The pain may increase, may not respond to a single nitroglycerin dose, and may persist for >5 minutes. Usually pain is more frequent, lasts longer, and may occur at rest when sitting or lying down. Unstable angina may indicate a rupture of an atherosclerotic plaque and the beginning of thrombus formation, so it should always be treated as a medical emergency with rapid transport because it may indicate a myocardial infarction. **Variant angina** (also known as Prinzmetal's angina) results from spasms of the coronary arteries; can be associated with or without atherosclerotic plaques; and is often related to smoking, alcohol, or illicit stimulants. Variant angina frequently occurs cyclically at the same time each day and often while the person is at rest. Nitroglycerin or calcium channel blockers are used for treatment. Prehospital: Provide supportive care and oxygen, and assist the patient to take nitroglycerin if available.

MYOCARDIAL INFARCTION (MI—HEART ATTACK)

Myocardial infarction (MI—heart attack) may occur after an episode of unstable angina caused by a rupture of an atherosclerotic plaque and thrombosis associated with coronary artery spasm, but it may also result from vasoconstriction, acute blood loss, decreased oxygen, and ingestion of cocaine. Symptoms may vary considerably, with males having the more "classic" symptom of a sudden onset of crushing chest pain. Elderly and diabetic patients may complain primarily of weakness. Symptoms include the following:

- Angina with pain in the chest that may radiate to the neck or arms, crushing pain, tightness (often more than 30 minutes and unrelieved by rest or nitroglycerin).
- Hypertension or hypotension.
- Palpitations, tachycardia, bradycardia, and dysrhythmias.
- Dyspnea.
- ECG changes (ST segment and T-wave changes), tachycardia, bradycardia, and dysrhythmias.
- Pulmonary edema, peripheral edema, weak/absent peripheral pulses.
- Nausea and vomiting.
- Pallor, cold and clammy skin, diaphoresis.
- Neurological/psychological disturbances: Anxiety, light-headedness, headache, visual abnormalities, slurred speech, and fear.

Prehospital: Manage the patient's airway/ventilation/oxygen supplementation, provide supportive care, perform CPR/defibrillation if needed, and provide rapid transport.

HEART FAILURE

Heart failure (HF, aka congestive HF) includes disorders of contractions (systolic "left-sided" dysfunction) or filling (diastolic dysfunction) or both, which result in hypertrophy (thickening, enlarging, and stiffening) of the myocardium (heart muscle). The most common causes are coronary artery disease, myocardial infarction, systemic or pulmonary hypertension, cardiomyopathy, and valvular disorders. Incidence of HF correlates with age. Left-sided HF may cause pulmonary edema that impairs ventilation, leading to hypoxia, especially when the patient is lying in a supine position, and right-sided HF may cause abdominal and peripheral edema of the feet and legs. The circulatory time with HF decreases overall, so changes in oximetry to show hypoxia may be delayed. The autonomic nervous system's regulation of breathing to control oxygen levels may be impaired, resulting in periodic breathing patterns, Cheyne-Stokes breathing, or central sleep apnea. Medications used to treat HF include ACE inhibitors (captopril, lisinopril), angiotensin receptor blockers (ARBs) (losartan, valsartan), beta-blockers (metoprolol, carvedilol), aldosterone agonists (spironolactone), and diuretics (hydrochlorothiazide, furosemide).

CHRONIC VERSUS ACUTE HEART FAILURE

Chronic heart failure develops insidiously over time as the heart muscles weaken and enlarge, so initially patients may only note fatigue, weight gain, and swelling in their feet and ankles. **Acute heart failure** is characterized by impairment of gas exchange and decreased cardiac output because of changes in preload, contractibility, and heart rhythm; symptoms are more acute and may include irregular heartbeat, chest pain, cough, and rapid breathing, wheezing, and cyanosis from lack of adequate oxygen. Patients may also suffer from anxiety, decreased activity tolerance, and disturbances in sleep patterns. Medical management is aimed at increasing cardiac function, providing support, and monitoring treatment. Patients often are acutely short of breath and sitting upright, with rales evident in their lungs. Assessment includes conducting primary and secondary surveys; taking a complete medical history including medication use/home oxygen use; and assessing the patient's level of consciousness, airway status (cough, sputum, labored breathing, tripod position), heart rate/rhythm, peripheral pulses, edema (pitting/nonpitting, ascites, sacral), and complications. Prehospital: Manage the patient's airway/ventilation/oxygen supplementation with a nonrebreather mask or BVM with high-flow oxygen, position for comfort, and suction if necessary.

THROMBOEMBOLISM AND PULMONARY EMBOLISM

Thromboembolism includes the formation of a thrombus (such as in the heart with atrial fibrillation and in the deep veins with immobilization) and an embolism in which a clot breaks off and travels through the circulatory system. Although thromboembolism may cause a heart attack or stroke, the most common presentation is a **pulmonary embolism (PE)** resulting from deep vein thrombosis. The patient may or may not complain of pain at the thrombus site, which may be swollen and erythematous (red), typically in a lower extremity. When the patient develops PE, the usual presentation is acute onset of dyspnea and tachycardia and sitting in the tripod position. Some patients may have ECG abnormalities, frothy sputum, cough, fever, hemoptysis, and jugular vein distension. Prehospital: Provide supportive care; manage the patient's airway/ventilation/intubation as needed with oxygen to maintain oxygen saturation >94%.

CARDIAC TAMPONADE

Cardiac tamponade occurs when fluid, usually blood, accumulates in the pericardial sac. If the fluid accumulates rapidly, the walls of the pericardial sac do not have time to stretch to accommodate the fluid, so the patient may quickly develop pulseless electrical activity (PEA) with fluid accumulation of 50 to 250 mL. If fluid accumulates slowly, such as with pericardial effusions associated with cancer, patients may tolerate up to 2 L of fluid before symptoms become acute. Cardiac tamponade compresses the heart and limits the venous return to the heart and blood flow into the ventricles, thereby reducing cardiac output. Symptoms: Beck's triad includes decreased arterial BP, increased jugular venous distension, and muffled heart sounds. Patients may be anxious, dyspneic, dizzy, and have angina-like pain. Prehospital: Manage airway/high concentration oxygen, monitor the ECG, install an IV access line and give fluids as indicated, and provide rapid transport for pericardiocentesis.

JUGULAR VENOUS PRESSURE

Jugular venous pressure (neck vein) is used to assess the cardiac output and pressure in the right heart because the pulsations relate to changes in pressure in the right atrium. This procedure is usually not accurate if the pulse rate is >100. This is a noninvasive estimation of the central venous pressure and waveform. Measurement should be done with the internal jugular if possible; otherwise, the external jugular may be used.

- Elevate the patient's head to 45° (and to 90° if necessary) with the patient's head turned to the opposite side of examination.
- Position the light at an angle to illuminate the veins and shadows.
- Measure the height of the jugular vein pulsation above the sternal joint, using a ruler.
- The normal height of the jugular vein pulsation is ≤4 cm above the sternal angle.

Increased height (>4 cm) indicates increased pressure in the right atrium and right heart failure. It may also indicate pericarditis or tricuspid stenosis. Laughing or coughing may trigger the Valsalva response and also cause a pressure increase.

POISONING

Ingestion	Drugs, overdose, toxic/caustic liquids (bleach, cleaning solution, antifreeze, gasoline), mouse/rat poison, pesticides, some plants, and alcohol	Wide range of symptoms, depending on the substance: anaphylaxis, lethargy, constricted pupils, mouth burns, nausea and vomiting, pain, diarrhea, difficulty breathing, confusion, seizures, and coma. (Toddlers are particularly at risk.)

Inhalation	Toxic gases, smoke, hair spray, carbon monoxide, chlorine, halogens	Difficulty breathing, lethargy, confusion, nausea, vomiting, headache, cyanosis, seizures, slurred speech, and coma.
Injection	Heroin, morphine, drug overdose	Local irritation, lethargy, confusion, slurred speech, nausea, vomiting, difficulty breathing, seizures, and coma. (Adolescents are prone to experimentation with drugs.)
Absorption	Cleaning products, various chemicals	Local irritation, anaphylaxis, burns, tissue damage, rash, nausea, vomiting, shortness of breath, and confusion.

Prehospital: Treatment varies according to the severity. Contact a poison control center if necessary, provide supportive care, remove the substance residue from the patient's mouth, place the patient in the recovery position, manage the patient's airway/ventilation/oxygen supplementation, provide CPR as necessary, induce vomiting or administer activated charcoal only if advised by the poison control center or another expert, and provide rapid transport. If the contamination is by inhalation, remove patient from the source as soon as possible. If the contamination is by absorption, remove the contaminated clothes and wash the patient's skin with large amounts of soap and water and flush the affected eyes with water or NS.

Nerve Agents/Cholinergics

Nerve agents/Cholinergics are toxic chemicals (organophosphates) that damage the nervous system and bodily functions, leading to death in a short time. Nerve agents include tabun (GA), sarin (GB), soman (GD), and VX, and they are used in terrorist attacks. GA, BG, and GD persist in the environment for 10 minutes to 24 hours during the summer and 2 hours to 3 days during the winter (cold weather), and they have very fast action. VX persists longer in the environment and is more lethal. Symptoms of exposure (gas/aerosol) include salivation, lacrimation, urination, defecation, GI upset, and emesis (SLUDGE); runny nose; pupil contraction; vision impairment; slurred speech; chest pain; hallucinations; respiratory distress; and coma. High doses may cause immediate seizures and death. Prehospital: Move away from the area quickly or shelter in place, remove the patient's clothing, and wash the patient's body with large amounts of soap and water. Use an autoinjector for atropine and pralidoxime (separate injections [Mark I] or combined dose [DuoDote]), unless there is only mild tearing or a runny nose, and use diazepam for seizures. Provide airway/ventilation/oxygen supplementation and circulation support.

Carbon Monoxide Poisoning

Carbon monoxide poisoning occurs when people breathe in carbon monoxide, usually related to industrial or household accidents or suicide attempts. Carbon monoxide binds to hemoglobin 200 times more readily than oxygen, and once the carbon monoxide binds to hemoglobin (creating carboxyhemoglobin), the hemoglobin can no longer bind to or transport oxygen, resulting in hypoxemia. Symptoms vary depending on the percentage of saturation with carbon monoxide. At 10%, patients may complain of headache and nausea. At >20%, a patient becomes increasingly weak and confused with alterations in mental status. At >30%, a patient may have dyspnea, chest pain, and increased confusion. When the level continues to increase, a patient may experience seizures, coma, and death. The patient's skin color may be cyanotic, pink, or bright cherry red (but this is not a reliable sign). Prehospital: Administer 100% oxygen with a nonrebreather mask and transport.

Poison Control Resources

The **National Capital Poison Center** provides a website with an online tool—webPOISONCONTROL—(https://triage.webpoisoncontrol.org/#/exclusions) and a telephone number (1-800-222-1222) for people who swallow or come into contact (absorbed, inhaled, injected) with poisonous (toxic) substances.

- webPOISONCONTROL: Can be used for patients (ages 6 months to 79 years and nonpregnant women) who are asymptomatic and unintentionally swallowed a single drug or medication, household product, or berries over a short period of time (minutes to a few hours) and are otherwise healthy.
- Telephone contact: Is used for all other situations, including a patient with symptoms, pregnant women, nonswallowing contact, those ages <6 months or >79, or those who swallowed materials or substances other than those listed for online assistance. Telephone contact can be made for any poisoning if it is preferred to online assistance.

This service is free and usually requires about 3 minutes for a response. When calling, be prepared to describe the substance (include the product name and dosage for medications), amount swallowed, age of patient, weight of patient, time since exposure, and the patient's ZIP Code and email address. If unsure of the amount of poison or the weight of the victim, estimates are acceptable.

Age-Related Concerns Related to Toxicology

Age-related concerns related to toxicology include the following:

- Toddlers are at risk of ingestion of toxic substances because their taste buds are not yet fully developed and this allows them to drink foul-tasting substances, such as cleaning supplies, which may be kept under a sink where a child has easy access if the cabinet is not secured. Household substances that pose a substantial risk include perfumes, cosmetics, and alcohol. Toddlers may also ingest unsecured medications.
- Adolescents, who often experiment with drugs and alcohol, are at risk from alcohol poisoning and overdose or severe reaction to illicit drugs. Additionally, adolescents often attempt suicide with acetaminophen (Tylenol), sometimes to gain attention, without realizing that it can cause liver failure and death even after resuscitation.
- Geriatric patients are most at risk from medication errors, such as taking the wrong medication, taking medications belonging to friends or family, or taking the wrong dose of a medication.

Autoinjectors

Autoinjectors are spring-loaded syringe/needle devices that contain preloaded doses of medication and can be easily administered by following the directions on the devices. Autoinjectors are available for nerve agent treatment for emergency medical personnel—Mark I and DuoDote.

- Atropine autoinjector: For symptoms of nerve damage (increases heart rate, dries secretions, dilates pupils, and reduces GI upset).
- Pralidoxime (2-PAM chloride) autoinjector: For symptoms of nerve damage, twitching, and difficulty breathing.
- Diazepam autoinjector: For convulsions associated with nerve agents.

Wear appropriate PPE, remove the safety cap, cleanse the skin with alcohol, and (holding the device perpendicular to the skin) apply firm pressure with the tip of the injector against the skin in the outer thigh until the device fires the needle into the muscle tissue (avoid jabbing). Then, hold the autoinjector in place for at least 10 seconds to ensure that the medication is completely injected. Carefully remove the needle from the skin. Avoid touching the needle, and do not attempt to recap it. Dispose of the intact device in a sharps container.

Substance Abuse

Many people with **substance abuse** (alcohol or drugs) are reluctant to disclose this information. Common agents include cannabis (marijuana), hallucinogens (LSD), stimulants (cocaine, methamphetamine), barbiturates (secobarbital [Seconal], amobarbital [Amytal]), sedatives (zolpidem [Ambien], eszopiclone [Lunesta]), hypnotics/benzodiazepines (alprazolam [Xanax], diazepam [Valium], lorazepam [Ativan]), and opiates (heroin, morphine, fentanyl, oxycodone, hydrocodone). A number of indicators are suggestive of substance abuse.

- Physical signs
    - Needle tracks on arms or legs
    - Burns on fingers or lips
    - Pupils abnormally dilated or constricted, eyes watery
    - Slurring of speech, slow speech
    - Lack of coordination, instability of gait
    - Tremors
    - Sniffing repeatedly, nasal irritation
    - Persistent cough
    - Weight loss
    - Dysrhythmias (abnormal pulse)
    - Pallor, puffiness of face
- Other signs
    - Odor of alcohol/marijuana on clothing or breath
    - Labile emotions, including mood swings, agitation, and anger
    - Inappropriate, impulsive, and/or risky behavior
    - Lying
    - Missing appointments
    - Difficulty concentrating/short-term memory loss, disoriented/confused
    - Blackouts
    - Insomnia or excessive sleeping
    - Lack of personal hygiene

Ethanol (Alcohol) Abuse and Withdrawal

Ethanol (alcohol that is found in alcoholic beverages, flavorings, and some medications) is a multisystem toxin and CNS depressant. It is often the drug of choice of teenagers, young adults, and those >60 years old. Ethanol overdose affects the CNS and other organs. If patients are easily aroused, they can usually safely sleep off the effects, but if a patient is semiconscious or unconscious, emergency medical treatment is needed. Young children frequently ingest alcohol in products such as perfumes and cleaning solutions, which are often more toxic than alcoholic beverages.

Infants/Young children	Teenagers/Adults
Seizures, coma, death	Altered mental status, coma, circulatory collapse, death
Respiratory depression and hypoxia	Hypotension, bradycardia with arrhythmias
Hypoglycemia (especially infants and toddlers)	Respiratory depression and hypoxia
	Cold, clammy skin or flushed skin
Hypothermia	Acute pancreatitis/abdominal pain

Chronic abuse of ethanol (alcoholism) is associated with alcohol withdrawal syndrome (delirium tremens) with abrupt cessation of alcohol intake, resulting in hallucinations, tachycardia, diaphoresis, sometimes psychotic behavior, and a high mortality rate. Prehospital: Manage the patient's airway/ventilation/oxygen supplementation and provide CPR if necessary, maintain body temperature, and reduce noise/light.

Nonnarcotic Medication Overdose

Drug	Overdose symptoms
Acetaminophen (Tylenol)	Toxicity occurs with dosage >140 mg/kg in one dose or >7.5g in 24 hours: (Initial) Minor gastrointestinal upset. (Days 2–3) Hepatotoxicity (liver damage) with right upper quadrant pain. (Days 3–4) Hepatic failure with metabolic acidosis, coagulopathy, kidney failure, encephalopathy, nausea, vomiting, and possible death. (Days 5–12) Recovery period (survivors). Prehospital: Manage the patient's airway/ventilation/oxygen supplementation. Use the recovery position if the patient is nauseated. Provide supportive care.
NSAIDs/Salicylates	Toxicity (4 to 48 hours after ingestion) includes headache, nausea, abdominal pain, tinnitus (ringing in the ears), diaphoresis, hypertension, fluid in the lungs, alterations in mental status, cardiac dysrhythmias, seizures, and respiratory arrest. Prehospital: As above.
Dextromethorphan (cough syrup/cold medications)	Mild: Restlessness and euphoria and signs of intoxication. Moderate: Slurred speech, lack of coordination, memory loss, hallucinations, and "stoned" appearance. Severe: Altered state of consciousness, impaired vision, hearing, emotional detachment, inability to comprehend spoken words, leading to hallucinations, delusions, tachycardia, temporary blindness, and respiratory arrest. Some people exhibit violent or psychotic behavior. Prehospital: As above; restrain if necessary.
Cardiac	Digitalis (digoxin) toxicity may cause (initially) increasing fatigue, lethargy, depression, nausea, "halo" vision, and vomiting progressing to sudden changes in heart rhythm, such as an irregular rhythm, palpitations, heart block, tachycardia, and, later, bradycardia. Prehospital: Manage the patient's airway/ventilation/oxygen supplementation and circulation as needed.
Psychiatric	Benzodiazepine toxicity may result from accidental or intentional overdose with such drugs as Xanax and Valium. Indications are often nonspecific neurological changes such as lethargy, dizziness, alterations in consciousness, and ataxia. Respiratory depression and hypotension are rare complications. Prehospital: Provide supportive care. Mild lithium toxicity (Eskalith, Lithobid) can include severe vomiting and diarrhea, increased muscle tremors and twitching, lethargy, body aches, ataxia, ringing in the ears, blurry vision, vertigo, or hyperactive deep-tendon reflexes. More severe symptoms can include elevated temperature, low urine output, hypotension, heart abnormalities, decreased level of consciousness, seizures, coma, or death. Prehospital: Manage the patient's airway/ventilation/oxygen supplementation and circulation as needed.

Narcotics

Narcotics include opiates (drugs derived from opium) and opioids (synthetic narcotics). Drugs frequently abused include heroin and many prescription drugs such as morphine, meperidine, fentanyl (pills and patches), oxycodone, hydrocodone, buprenorphine, and methadone. Patients often crush pills and snort or inject them to increase the effects. Because tolerance to the drugs occurs, patients tend to take higher and higher doses, resulting in addiction and an increasing risk of overdose. Narcotics reduce pain and provide a feeling of euphoria or well-being as well as drowsiness. Symptoms of overdose may include slurred speech, pupil (pinpoint) constriction, nausea, hypotension, vomiting, lack of coordination, alterations of consciousness, coma, respiratory depression, cyanosis, and cardiac arrest (death). Patients may have a runny, irritated nose from snorting drugs or may have needle marks from injecting. Prehospital: Manage the patient's airway/ventilation/oxygen supplementation, and provide CPR if necessary. Administer naloxone (an opioid reversal agent) per autoinjector or nasal spray if protocol allows.

SPONTANEOUS PNEUMOTHORAX

Spontaneous pneumothorax is air in the pleural space that causes the lung to collapse but without an obvious cause. Symptoms include an abrupt onset of sharp chest pain on the affected side, dyspnea, difficulty breathing, and decreased/absent respirations on the affected side.

- Primary (no underlying lung disease): It is most common in tall, thin adolescents and young adults and is associated with cigarette smoking. Often resolves without treatment and rarely progresses to tension pneumothorax.
- Secondary (underlying lung disease): It is most common in those with chronic obstructive pulmonary disease (COPD), cystic fibrosis, and severe asthma, and it poses a risk of death because of respiratory compromise. Patients may develop hypoxemia, altered mental status, coma, and tension pneumothorax.

Prehospital: Manage the patient's airway/ventilation/oxygen supplementation, place the patient in a position of comfort, and transport. A large spontaneous pneumothorax will require catheter aspiration of air or insertion of a chest tube.

EPIGLOTTITIS

Acute epiglottitis (supraglottitis) occurs in children primarily from 1 to 8 years old and in young adults. Acute epiglottitis requires immediate medical attention because it can rapidly become obstructive. The onset is usually very sudden and often occurs during the night. The patient may awaken suddenly with a fever, but he or she usually does not have a cough. Symptoms include:

- Tripod position: Sits upright, leaning forward, mouth open, and tongue protruding.
- Agitation: Appears restless, tense, and agitated.
- Drooling: Excess secretions combined with pain or dysphagia and a mouth-open position.
- Voice: No hoarseness, but his or her voice sounds thick and "froglike."
- Cyanosis: Color is usually pale and sallow initially but may progress to frank cyanosis.
- Throat: On examination, the epiglottis appears bright red and swollen. Note: The patient's throat should not be examined with a tongue blade unless intubation and tracheostomy equipment is immediately available because the examination can trigger an obstruction.

Prehospital: Provide rapid transport, administer high-flow oxygen with blow-by mask, or provide slow ventilation with a BVM.

RESPIRATORY CONDITIONS

Respiratory condition	Assessment/Findings	Prehospital
Asthma	An immune response causes constriction of bronchi and inflammation and increased secretions in the lower airways. Symptoms include cough, wheezing, diminished breath sounds, and dyspnea.	Assist with albuterol (nebulized/metered dose) and oxygen (6–8 LPM), and provide airway management/ventilation. Provide CPAP for moderate/severe cases. Severe: Provide rapid transport.
Pulmonary edema	Often secondary to congestive heart failure or pulmonary embolus, fluid collects in the lung alveoli (air sacs), resulting in severe shortness of breath, wheezing, rapid pulse, cough, and chest pain.	Place the patient in a position of comfort (usually with head elevated), manage the patient's airway/ventilation, and provide supplemental oxygen. Severe: Provide rapid transport.

Respiratory condition	Assessment/Findings	Prehospital
Pneumonia	Infection of the lungs (bacterial, viral, fungal, or parasitic) resulting in fever, chills, cough, purulent sputum, and difficulty breathing, chest pain on cough or deep inhalation, and headache. Infants may exhibit sternal retraction, decreased feeding, and irritability. Adolescents may have vomiting, diarrhea, sore throat, and earache along with typical symptoms.	Use standard and droplet precautions, including wearing a protective face mask. Place the patient in a position of comfort (usually with the head elevated), and manage the patient's airway/ventilation/oxygen supplementation. Severe: Provide rapid transport.
Pertussis (whooping cough)	Severe persistent "whooping" cough, thick sputum, postcough emesis, petechiae on the upper body, and sclera from exertion. Infants may develop CNS damage, apnea, or pneumonia; children may develop hernia or muscle damage; and adults may develop hernia or a fractured rib.	Use standard and droplet precautions, provide the patient a position of comfort, and manage the patient's airway/ventilation/oxygen supplementation as needed.
Cystic fibrosis	Progressive congenital disease that particularly affects the pancreas and lungs, causing the production of thick mucus that clogs the lungs and causes recurrent bacterial infections. Symptoms include severe cough, sputum, fever, and dyspnea.	Use standard and droplet precautions, and provide the patient a position of comfort. Manage the patient's airway/ventilation/oxygen supplementation. Severe: Provide rapid transport.
Chronic obstructive pulmonary disease (COPD)	Disease with limitations of airflow, narrowing airways, exertional dyspnea, chronic cough, right-sided heart failure (cor pulmonale), damaged, distended alveoli, and barrel chest. Symptoms include severe dyspnea, cough, and the tripod position.	Manage the patient's airway/ventilation, and provide oxygen per nonrebreather mask to maintain oxygen saturation >90%. Provide the patient a position of comfort. Severe: Provide rapid transport.

PULMONARY EDEMA

Pulmonary edema occurs when the alveoli in the lungs fill with fluid.

- Cardiogenic: The left ventricle weakens, so the heart cannot pump adequate amounts of blood, resulting in back pressure in the left atrium and the vessels in the lungs, forcing fluid into the alveoli. Left ventricular damage can result from coronary artery disease, cardiomyopathy, myocardial infarction, defective heart valves, and uncontrolled hypertension.
- Noncardiogenic: Damage to the capillaries in the lungs causes them to leak fluid into the alveoli. Conditions causing noncardiogenic pulmonary edema include acute respiratory distress syndrome (ARDS), adverse drug reactions, pulmonary embolism, lung injury, viral infections, nervous system conditions, toxin exposure, smoke inhalation, near drowning, and high-altitude pulmonary edema (HAPE).

Symptoms include severe dyspnea, orthopnea, tachycardia, cough, and chest pain. Prehospital: Manage airway/ventilation and supplemental oxygen/CPAP or intubation with PEEP, and start an IV access line. Medications may include dopamine, dobutamine, nitroglycerin, and furosemide (per protocol). Severe cases require rapid transport. HAPE: Immediately descend to a lower altitude (500–1000 m), provide supplemental oxygen and a portable hyperbaric chamber, and administer acetazolamide or dexamethasone (per protocol).

METERED-DOSE INHALER (MIDI/MDI) AND THE SMALL-VOLUME NEBULIZER

The AEMT may assist the patient with use of a metered-dose inhaler (MIDI/MDI) or a small-volume nebulizer for medications such as albuterol, according to protocol as follows:

- The **MIDI/MDI** is a pressurized cartridge that is used for administration of a specific dose of an aerosolized medication. Shake the medication vigorously before use, prime if it is the initial use, position 4 cm (two finger widths) away from the patient's mouth or between the lips, have the patient exhale and breathe in slowly and completely while the MIDI is activated, and then have the patient hold the breath for 10 seconds, waiting 1 minute between puffs. Stop the treatment if the patient becomes shaky, dizzy, coughs uncontrollably, has palpitations, or has a pulse increase of ≥20 bpm. Resume slowly after 5 to 10 minutes.
- A **small-volume nebulizer** includes a nebulizer cup that holds 2 to 4 mL of medication, air tubing, a compressor to aerosolize the medication, and a T-piece and mouthpiece or face mask for delivery. Dilute the medication with sterile NS or water, not tap water, if necessary. Have the patient sit upright for treatment, breathing normally through the mouth and using the mouthpiece or face mask.

SICKLE CELL DISEASE

Sickle cell disease is a recessive genetic disorder of chromosome 11, causing hemoglobin to be defective so that the red blood cells (RBCs) are sickle-shaped and inflexible, resulting in their accumulating in small vessels and causing painful blockages. Although normal RBCs survive for 120 days, sickled blood cells may survive only 10–20 days, stressing the bone marrow that can't produce RBCs fast enough and resulting in anemia. Different types of **crises** occur (aplastic, hemolytic, vaso-occlusive, and sequestering), which can cause infarctions in organs, severe pain, damage to organs, and rapid enlargement of the liver and spleen. Vaso-occlusive crisis is common in adolescents and adults, and it can be triggered by sickness, stress, dehydration, temperature changes, and high altitude. Young children are prone to splenic sequestration (RBCs trapped in the spleen, causing it to enlarge and sometimes rupture), which is characterized by pain in the left abdomen. Prehospital: Manage the patient's airway/ventilation/oxygen supplementation and circulation, provide emotional support, and provide rapid transport for severe symptoms.

CLOTTING DISORDERS

Clotting disorders include the following:

- Hemophilia is an inherited disorder in which the person lacks adequate clotting factors, which results in bleeding with trauma, bruising, spontaneous hemorrhage (often in the joints), and epistaxis. There are three primary types: A (80%–90%), B, and C.
- Disseminated intravascular coagulation (DIC) (consumption coagulopathy) is a secondary disorder that is triggered by another event, such as trauma, congenital heart disease, necrotizing enterocolitis, sepsis, and severe viral infections. DIC triggers coagulation (clotting) and hemorrhage through a complex series of events, with clotting and hemorrhage occurring simultaneously, putting the patient at risk of death.
- Von Willebrand's disease is a group of congenital bleeding disorders (inherited from either parent) affecting 1%–2% of the population, associated with deficiency or lack of von Willebrand factor (vWF), a glycoprotein.

Prehospital: Monitor for signs of bleeding, and manage the patient's airway/ventilation/oxygen supplementation. Provide rapid transport for hemorrhage or acute blood loss resulting in hypotension.

HEMODIALYSIS

Hemodialysis is used primarily for those who have progressed from renal insufficiency to uremia with end-stage renal (kidney) disease (ESRD). With hemodialysis, blood is circulated outside of the body through a dialyzer (a synthetic semipermeable membrane), which filters the blood and removes waste products and excess fluids. A vascular access device, such as a catheter, fistula, or graft must be established for hemodialysis

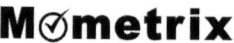

with fistulas and grafts usually being placed in an arm and a catheter being placed in the upper chest (into the superior vena cava). Tubing from the dialysis machine attaches to the access device for treatments, which are usually done for 4 hours three times weekly. Emergent conditions include low BP, nausea/vomiting, irregular pulse, cardiac arrest, bleeding from the access site, and difficulty breathing. Missed treatments may result in electrolyte excess, weakness, and pulmonary edema. Prehospital: Manage the patient's airway/ventilation/oxygen supplementation, apply pressure to stop any bleeding, position the patient flat if he or she is in shock, and position him or her upright if having difficulty breathing.

PERITONEAL DIALYSIS

Peritoneal dialysis is used to remove waste products and excess fluids from those with ESRD. A catheter is placed into the peritoneal cavity of the abdomen. The peritoneum comprises the visceral peritoneum (the lining of the gut and other viscera), which makes up about 80% of the total peritoneal surface area, and the parietal perineum (lining the abdominal cavity), which is the most important for peritoneal dialysis. A dialysate solution is instilled (usually about 2 L for adults but less for children, taking about 10 minutes) through the catheter, the catheter is clamped, and the solution (dwell) is left in place for 3–6 hours. The solution is then drained (usually for about 20 minutes), and the process is repeated with new dialysate. Peritoneal dialysis increases the risk of obesity, peritonitis, hernia, malnutrition, hypertriglyceridemia, and back pain. Obesity, older adulthood, and lack of social support are contraindications for peritoneal dialysis. Prehospital: Manage the patient's airway/ventilation/oxygen supplementation, use contact precautions if there is purulent drainage from catheter site, and position the patient for comfort.

URINARY CATHETER MANAGEMENT

A **urinary catheter** is inserted through the urethra and into the bladder to drain urine. Straight catheterizations are done with sterile catheters periodically to empty the bladder or to relieve urinary retention, whereas retention catheters (Foley) have a balloon that inflates to keep the catheter in place for continuous drainage. Foley catheters may be indicated for patients with neuromuscular disorders, incontinence, urinary retention, dementia, or urinary disorders. Catheters may also be inserted suprapubically (above the pubis bone) directly into the bladder, especially for males with long-term catheterization. Urinary collection bags should be kept below the level of the bladder, and the tubing is secured so that the catheter is not inadvertently pulled out, causing trauma to the urethra, especially in males. Thick, cloudy urine may indicate infection. Scant urine and lower abdominal pain/distension may indicate blockage of the catheter. Milking the catheter may help relieve a blockage. When removing a Foley catheter, the balloon must first be deflated. Prehospital: Provide supportive care.

RENAL CALCULI

Renal (kidney) and urinary calculi (stones) occur frequently, more commonly in males, and they can relate to diseases (hyperparathyroidism, renal tubular acidosis, and gout) and lifestyle factors, such as sedentary work. Their incidence is highest between ages 35 and 45. Additionally, some medications can precipitate calculi. Calculi can form at any age, most are composed of calcium, and they can range in size from very tiny to >6mm. Stones of <4mm can usually pass in the urine easily.

Symptoms	Prehospital
Symptoms occur with obstruction and are usually of sudden onset and acute. Severe flank pain radiating to abdomen and labia or testicle on the same side as the stone (adolescents and adults), abdominal or pelvic pain (young children) Nausea and vomiting Diaphoresis Hematuria (blood in urine)	Analgesia: Opiates and NSAIDs as needed (per protocol) Provide supplemental oxygen if needed Start an IV access line and give fluids if indicated Transport

Renal (Kidney) Failure

Acute renal (kidney) failure is abrupt and is an almost complete failure of kidney function, occurring over a period of hours/days. It most commonly occurs in hospitalized patients, but it may occur in others as well. Causes include myocardial infarction, heart failure, sepsis, anaphylaxis, burns, trauma, infections, transfusion reactions, medications (NSAIDs and ACE inhibitors), and obstruction. **Chronic liver failure** occurs after years of disease that damages the kidneys, often being essentially asymptomatic until the damage is severe. Prehospital: Manage the patient's airway/ventilation/oxygen, provide an IV access line (if the patient is hypotensive or if there is evidence of pulmonary edema), and transport.

End-Stage Renal Disease (ESRD)

Acute and chronic liver failure may progress to **end-stage renal disease (ESRD)** when the kidneys are no longer able to function and the patient needs dialysis or a kidney transplant. The patient may develop uremic syndrome, which results in decreased production of red blood cells and platelets, electrolyte imbalances, bone disease, multiple endocrine disorders, cardiac problems (especially congestive heart failure), anorexia, and malnutrition. Symptoms include altered mental status, hallucinations, and confusion from the accumulation of waste products in the blood; increasing edema and shortness of breath from accumulated fluids; chest and bone pain; severe pruritus; nausea, vomiting, and diarrhea; tremors, muscle twitching, and seizures; and increased bruising and discoloration of the skin. Prehospital: Manage the patient's airway/ventilation/oxygen, start an IV access line (if the patient is hypotensive or if there is evidence of pulmonary edema), and transport.

Vaginal Bleeding

Vaginal bleeding may indicate heavy menstrual bleeding (menorrhagia) or abnormal bleeding between cycles (metrorrhagia). Vaginal bleeding may also be an indication of an ectopic pregnancy or spontaneous abortion; in postmenopausal women, it may be a sign of endometrial cancer. Menorrhagia may result from hormonal imbalance, clotting disorders, uterine fibroids, and endometrial polyps. Metrorrhagia may result from infection, cancer, and cervical/endometrial polyps. Symptoms may include cramping and abdominal pain, depending on the cause. It's important to determine when the bleeding started and about how much blood had been lost (the number of sanitary pads that are saturated per hour, for example) as well as the presence or absence of pain. If blood loss is excessive, the patient may exhibit signs of shock. Prehospital: Use standard precautions, manage the patient's airway/ventilation/oxygen supplementation. Monitor vital signs. Position the patient flat for shock, and provide IV access and fluids.

Female Reproductive System

The **female reproductive system** includes the ovaries, fallopian tubes, uterus, cervix, vagina, vulva, labia minora, labia majora, clitoris, and breasts. Functions include ovulation, fertilization, menstruation, pregnancy, and lactation. Menarche (onset of menses) is usually between 9 and 15, but it may occur in younger girls and should be considered as a possibility with younger girls. Menopause occurs at approximately age 50, usually following a period of about 10 years of irregular periods during which time the person may become pregnant. The normal menstrual cycle is 28 days, but it may be up to 45 days in adolescents. Assessment should include abdominal or vaginal pain, vaginal bleeding or discharge, fever, nausea and vomiting, and dizziness. Patients should have their privacy protected during an examination, and the AEMT should communicate openly, asking for permission to touch the patient. The AEMT should consider the possibility of pregnancy or sexually transmitted disease with any abnormal condition.

> **Review Video: Reproductive Systems**
> Visit mometrix.com/academy and enter code: 505450

Sexual Assault

The crime scenes associated with a **sexual assault** include the patient (body, injuries, clothing, and emotional response) and the place the assault occurred. A victim of sexual assault has the right to consent to or refuse each element of a sexual assault evaluation, although some states may mandate reporting of sexual assault to the authorities. The AEMT should wear disposable gloves when handling clothing, and clothing should be handled gently so that evidence, such as strands of hair or other materials, is not lost in transfer. Documenting the assault should be done in detail with direct quotations. If the patient refuses transport, the best approach is to point out services that could benefit the patient, such as prophylaxis to prevent STDs and pregnancy. Patients are often frightened and confused, so pressuring them to protect others or trying to frighten them more by suggesting that they might be pregnant or develop an STD is a negative approach that may backfire.

SEXUALLY TRANSMITTED DISEASES

Disease	Characteristics/Considerations
Gonorrhea	Caused by the bacterial species *Neisseria gonorrhoeae*. Transmission is through anal, oral, or vaginal sex. The incubation period is 3 to 8 days. Male symptoms include painful urination, purulent discharge from the penis, and swollen testicles. Females are asymptomatic, or they may have mild difficulty urinating. Complications include prostatitis, orchitis, epididymitis, and sterility (males) and pelvic inflammatory disease and disseminated disease (females). It is treated with antibiotics. The infection may pass to a newborn during birth, causing gonorrheal eye infection and blindness unless eye prophylaxis is provided. Prehospital: Use standard precautions.
Chlamydia	Caused by the bacterial species *Chlamydia trachomatis*. Transmission is through anal, oral, or vaginal sex. It often occurs with gonorrhea. Symptoms: Many are asymptomatic, but the disease can spread and cause urethritis, proctitis, and epididymitis (males) and painful intercourse, pelvic inflammatory disease, fallopian tube damage, and vaginal bleeding (females). Complications include sterility and infertility. Treatment is with antibiotics. Prehospital: Use standard precautions.
Syphilis (*Treponema pallidum*)	Bacterial infection transmitted through oral, anal, or vaginal sex and needle sharing. The incubation period is 10 to 90 days. Primary symptoms (3–8 weeks): Chancres (very contagious). Secondary symptoms (1–2 years): Flu-like symptoms and rash, weight loss, and hair loss. Latent symptoms (>2 years): Asymptomatic. Noncontagious after 4 years. Treatment is antibiotics. Late/Tertiary symptoms: Gummas (lesions) in multiple organs, heart abnormalities, CNS impairment with psychosis, confusion, ataxia, and difficulty speaking. Prehospital: Standard precautions.
Genital herpes (herpes simplex virus 2)	Transmitted though oral, anal, or vaginal sex. The virus enters nerve endings, travels to the nerve ganglion, and stays dormant until reactivated by stress, immunosuppression, menstruation, sunburn, illness, or other triggers. Initial symptoms: Small vesicular lesions in genital area that rupture and leave open crusting sores; painful urination; flu-like symptoms. Recurrent symptoms are less severe, lasting 8–12 days. Complications include dissemination to other areas of the body, aseptic meningitis, and damage to nerves resulting in atonic bladder, constipation, and impotence. Treatment is with antiviral agents. Prehospital: Use standard, contact, and airborne precautions until disseminated herpes is ruled out.

MUSCULOSKELETAL SYSTEM

The musculoskeletal system includes 206 bones including long bones (e.g., the femur in the thigh), short bones (e.g., the carpal bones in the fingers), and flat bones (e.g., the sternum). The outer hard shell of the bone is the cortex, and the inner porous area is the trabecular bone. The vertebrae lack the cortex layer. Long bones have three parts: The middle section is the diaphysis, followed by the metaphyses, and then the epiphyses (the bone ends). In growing children, an epiphyseal plate of cartilage separates the metaphyses and epiphyses, allowing bone growth. This closes in adults, but damage to this area in a child may impair bone growth. The middle part of the short bones contains yellow bone marrow (fatty tissue). Red bone marrow, which produces blood cells, is found in the middle of the flat bones (pelvis, sternum, ribs, and scapula) and at the ends (epiphyses) of long bones. The skeletal system is connected by cartilage and tendons, and it is protected, supported, and allowed movement by about 700 soft-tissue muscles.

NONTRAUMATIC FRACTURES

Nontraumatic fractures occur when the bone weakens and can no longer support the body, such as may occur with a cancerous tumor of the bone or osteoporosis. Common fractures associated with osteoporosis include fractures of the vertebrae and hip. Osteoporotic fractures are most common in older adults, but they may also occur in adolescents with eating disorders. Infants and young children with multiple nontraumatic, nonabusive fractures may have a genetic disorder, such as osteogenesis imperfecta. Assessment of suspected fractures includes evaluating pain/tenderness, swelling around the fracture site, loss of sensation or movement, circulatory impairment (note the color of the skin, pallor or cyanosis), and deformity (especially noticeable in limb fractures). Prehospital: Splint extremity fractures; manage the patient's airway/ventilation/oxygen supplementation as needed; and provide transport for treatment.

NOSEBLEED (EPISTAXIS)

Recurrent **nosebleed (epistaxis)** is common in young children (2–10), especially boys, and it is often related to nose picking, dry climate, trauma, or central heating. Incidence also increases between 50–80 years of age and may be associated with nonsteroidal anti-inflammatory drugs (NSAIDs), hypertension, and anticoagulants. Patients abusing cocaine may suffer nosebleeds because of damage to the mucosa. The anterior (front) nares have plentiful blood vessels and bleed easily, usually from one nostril. Bleeding in the posterior (back) nares is more dangerous and can result in considerable blood loss. Blood may flow through both nostrils or backward into the throat, and the person may be observed swallowing and may vomit blood. The blood may block the airway in unconscious patients. Prehospital: Sit the patient in an upright position, leaning forward so the blood doesn't flow down the throat if the patient is conscious; pinch nostrils together firmly for at least 10 minutes; and advise the patient to avoid sniffing or blowing the nose.

Shock and Resuscitation

SHOCK

Shock is a life-threatening condition that occurs when the tissues do not receive adequate oxygen, such as with severe bleeding or fluid loss, severe infection, heart failure, or abnormal dilation of the blood vessels. Signs/Symptoms of shock include the following: extreme thirst; anxiety and restlessness; weak, rapid pulse; altered mental status progressing to loss of consciousness; rapid, shallow respirations; hypotension (low BP—often a late sign); and cool, clammy, pale skin with mottling sometimes on extremities from inadequate perfusion. If left untreated, shock may lead to cardiac arrest. Note that geriatric patients may have a higher baseline respiration and heart rate and irregular pulse. Prehospital: Request the assistance of advanced EMS if necessary, apply pressure to control the bleeding, perform spinal stabilization if needed, place the patient in the shock position (flat with feet elevated above the level of the heart, 8 to 12 inches), manage the patient's airway/ventilation and administer high-concentration oxygen, provide warming blankets to maintain body temperature, and provide reassurance. Provide rapid transport if needed. **Shock** generally occurs in stages as the body tries to compensate: Compensated shock occurs in the early stage while the body speeds up the heart rate and respirations and diverts blood to the vital organs (resulting in pale, cool skin) to maintain adequate perfusion and BP. Decompensated shock occurs when the body can no longer compensate and the BP falls and symptoms worsen. With irreversible shock, recovery is no longer possible because of cell damage caused by inadequate oxygenation and perfusion. Types of shock include the following:

Type of shock	Cause
Cardiogenic	Heart failure, myocardial infarction, drug overdose, dysrhythmia, congenital heart disease.
Distributive	Anaphylaxis, drug overdose.
Hypovolemic	Hemorrhage, severe vomiting and/or diarrhea, severe burns, dehydration.
Obstructive	Pneumothorax, pericardial tamponade.
Neurogenic	Spinal cord injury (a form of distributive shock because of decreased vascular tone).
Septic	Sepsis, severe infections. (This is also a form of distributive shock.)

Signs and symptoms are similar for all types of shock even though the mechanisms are different.

RESPIRATORY FAILURE/ARREST

Respiratory failure occurs when ventilation is insufficient for adequate gas exchange so that levels of carbon dioxide in the blood increase and levels of oxygen decrease. Respiratory failure may result from respiratory infection (pneumonia, tuberculosis), heart failure, chronic respiratory illness (asthma, chronic bronchitis, COPD), trauma, and depression of the central nervous system (usually from medications or trauma). Respiratory failure may be acute with sudden onset or chronic, developing over time. If untreated, respiratory failure can lead to **respiratory arrest**, which in turn leads to cardiac arrest. Indications of respiratory failure include altered mental status, cyanosis, labored breathing (dyspnea and orthopnea), coughing, fatigue, diminished breath sounds, and the presence of rales (crackles) and rhonchi (snoring/whistling sound). Patients may have hemoptysis (bloody sputum). The patient's oxygen saturation level is lower than 90% per pulse oximeter. Prehospital: Manage the patient's airway/ventilation/oxygen supplementation; positive-pressure ventilation may be needed. Place the patient in a position of comfort (usually high Fowler's).

POST-RESUSCITATION RETURN OF SPONTANEOUS CIRCULATION (ROSC)

If a patient undergoing resuscitation has **return of spontaneous circulation (ROSC)**, the patient's ventilation and oxygenation must be supported to maintain oxygen saturation ≥94% but below 100% to avoid hyperoxia. Ventilation should be maintained at 10–12 breaths per minute with an $ETCO_2$ value at 35–40 mm Hg. Hyperventilation must be avoided. Hypotension (systolic BP <90 mm Hg) should be treated with an IV bolus

(1–2 L saline) and vasopressor infusion. Treatable causes (the five H's and five T's) should be addressed, and a 12-lead ECG should be used to monitor the patient's condition. If the patient is nonresponsive, therapeutic hypothermia (to 32–24° C) for 12–24 hours may be considered as a neuroprotective measure. If the patient is responsive and able to follow commands, he or she should be immediately transported to the appropriate receiving facility: the ICU or cardiac cath lab for acute myocardial infarction (AMI) or ST-elevated myocardial infarction (STEMI) for percutaneous coronary intervention (PCI). Note: Brain damage begins within 4–6 minutes of cardiac arrest and is irreversible after 8–10 minutes.

Impedance Threshold Device (ITD)

The **impedance threshold device** (such as ResQPOD ITD) is a small, single-use device that fits into the airway circuit (face mask or advanced airway) with CPR. During CPR, compressions generate positive pressure that promotes cardiac output and, when released completely, negative pressure (vacuum) within the thorax that refills the heart, so adequate negative pressure ensures better filling. During compressions with the ITD, a valve in the device allows air to escape but, when the compressions are released, the valve closes to prevent the intake of air, increasing negative pressure and improving circulation on subsequent compressions; however, the device allows the paramedic to ventilate the patient, and the device has flashing timing lights every 6 seconds (so one ventilation with every flash equals 10 per minute). The ITD may double the blood flowing to the heart and double the systolic BP as well as increase cerebral perfusion.

Cardiopulmonary Resuscitation (CPR) for Cardiac Arrest

Cardiac arrest of unknown cause in adults or children is usually treated as though it were ventricular fibrillation or pulseless ventricular tachycardia, but the protocol varies. **Cardiopulmonary resuscitation (CPR)** involves the following components:

- Immediate defibrillation (one shock) is performed according to protocol with an AED/manual defibrillator (preferred) followed by CPR, beginning with compressions (30:2 compression to ventilation at the rate of 100–120 per minute at least 2 inches deep; two-finger compressions, to one-third of the chest depth for infants and children) for 2 minutes/five cycles and repeat defibrillation.
- Repeat cycles of 2 minutes CPR and defibrillation. (Laypeople may use compression-only CPR.)
- If a defibrillator is not readily available, CPR may begin first. Note that if a BVM is used, the break in compressions should not exceed 10 seconds. If an advanced airway/intubation is in place, ventilation should be at the rate of 8 to 10 per minute, maintaining oxygen saturation ≥94% but <100% with ventilation between compressions.
- The $ETCO_2$ value should be 10–20 mm Hg if chest compressions are adequate, increasing to 35 to 45 mm Hg with the return of spontaneous circulation (ROSC).

With **automated chest compression devices** for CPR, manual CPR should be started while the equipment is obtained and readied. These devices are only intended for adults and nontraumatic arrests, and they must be removed for defibrillation.

- Piston-driven device (Thumper): Uses pneumatic (air) power on a piston device set at a prescribed compression depth. The backboard must first be secured with straps, the device is slid into a slot in the backboard, the massager pad is placed over the sternum, the device is turned on, and the compression depth is then set. The device can also control ventilations and tidal volume.
- LUCAS device: It is also piston driven and is similar to the Thumper, but it applies decompression suction on recoil to increase negative pressure and it does not provide for ventilations.
- Load-distributing band/Vest CPR (AutoPulse): Device that contains a backboard and fits like a vest around the patient's chest and applies compression to the chest and about the thorax, increasing perfusion pressure. It can be set for continuous compressions or 30:2, and it automatically adjusts to the patient's size.

HEIMLICH MANEUVER

The universal sign of choking is when a person clutches his or her throat and appears to be choking or gasping for breath. If the person can speak ("Can you speak?") or cough, the **Heimlich maneuver** is not usually necessary. The Heimlich maneuver can be done with the victim sitting, standing, or supine. The Heimlich procedure for children (≥1 year) and adults is as follows:

- Wrap your arms around the victim's waist from the back if sitting or standing. Make a fist and place the thumb side against the victim's abdomen slightly above the umbilicus. Grasp this hand with the other and thrust sharply upward to force air out of the lungs.
- Repeat as needed.
- If the victim loses consciousness, ease him or her into a supine position on the floor, place your hands similarly to CPR but over the abdomen while sitting astride the victim's legs. Repeat upward compressions five times. If no ventilation occurs, attempt to sweep the mouth and ventilate the lungs mouth to mouth. Repeat compressions and ventilations until recovery.

Indications of choking in infants of less than 1 year include lack of breathing, gasping, cyanosis, and the inability to cry. The procedure for **Heimlich chest thrusts** includes the following:

- Position the infant in the prone (face-down) position along your forearm with the infant's head being lower than the trunk, being sure to support the head so the airway is not blocked.
- Using the heel of the hand, deliver five forceful upward blows between the shoulder blades.
- Sandwich the child between your two arms, and turn the infant into the supine position and drape over your thigh with his or her head lower than the trunk and the head supported.
- Using two fingers (as for CPR compressions), give up to five thrusts (about 1.5 inches deep) to the lower third of the sternum.
- Only do a finger sweep and remove a foreign object if the object is visible. Repeat five back blows, five chest thrusts until the foreign body is ejected.
- If the infant loses consciousness, begin CPR. If a pulse is noted but spontaneous respirations are absent, continue with ventilation only.

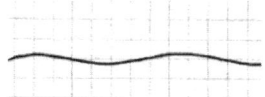

EMERGENCY DEFIBRILLATION WITH AN AUTOMATED EXTERNAL DEFIBRILLATOR (AED)

Emergency defibrillation is done for acute ventricular fibrillation or ventricular tachycardia with no audible or palpable pulse; it is ineffective for asystole or pulseless electrical activity. Defibrillation delivers an electrical discharge through paddles applied to both sides of the chest. **Automated external defibrillators (AEDs)** are frequently used by first responders, although manual defibrillators require less downtime from CPR. The procedure is as follows:

- Turn on the AED and apply pads to the chest (the position may vary according to the manufacturer). Infants and small children: If the pads touch, apply one to the chest and the back.
- Plug in the connector if necessary.
- Do not touch the patient while the AED analyzes the heart rhythm.
- Follow the directions for shocking, and warn others to stand clear.
- Continue CPR, beginning with compressions for 2 minutes/five cycles between defibrillations.
- If the patient is wet, wipe off his or her chest before applying the pads. Remove any transdermal patches on the chest, and shave excessive hair before applying the pads. If the patient has an implanted device, the pads should be placed at least 1 inch (2.5 cm) away.

Pulseless electrical activity is any rhythm without a palpable pulse (this is common after defibrillation). Identifying and correcting the underlying cause is critical for treatment. Common causes include:

- **Five H's**
    - Hypokalemia/Hyperkalemia
    - Hypoxia
    - Hypothermia
    - Hypovolemia
    - Hydrogen ion (acidosis)
- **Five T's**
    - Toxins
    - Tamponade (cardiac)
    - Tension pneumothorax
    - Thrombosis (lungs)
    - Thrombosis (heart)

Prehospital: Begin CPR, start an IV access line, administer epinephrine (per protocol) every 3 to 5 minutes, provide intubation and ventilation, and give oxygen as indicated. Provide rapid transport.

Asystole ("flatlined") is the absence of an audible heartbeat, palpable pulse, and respirations. The ECG may show some P waves initially. The QRS complex is absent, although there may be an occasional QRS "escape beat." Prehospital: Check the leads, begin CPR, start an IV access line, administer epinephrine every 3 to 5 minutes, provide intubation and ventilation, and give oxygen. Provide rapid transport.

ETHICAL ISSUES IN WITHHOLDING RESUSCITATION ATTEMPTS

Although the goal of EMS is to save lives, it is not always possible or ethical to carry out resuscitation efforts. **Withholding resuscitation** is justified under the following conditions:

- The patient's condition is not compatible with life (decapitation, crushed chest, severe open head injury with loss of brain tissue), and the patient is not breathing and has no pulse.
- The patient exhibits obvious signs of death, such as rigor mortis or livor mortis, indicating that he or she can no longer be resuscitated.
- The patient has a do-not-resuscitate (DNR) form available, and it is properly signed. Note: The AEMT cannot accept the word of family or friends that the patient does not want to be resuscitated without a DNR order.
- Conditions are unsafe to approach the patient and/or administer resuscitation efforts. This may occur, for example, if there are gunshots heard in the area, if the patient is pinned under a motor vehicle, or if the patient cannot safely be reached in time because of difficult terrain.

Trauma

BLUNT TRAUMA (NONBLEEDING)

Motor vehicle crashes	Result in 30%–40% of accidental deaths and half of closed-head and spinal cord injuries with injuries usually more serious with ejection, lateral (T-bone) impacts, and unrestrained patients, although lap belts increase the risk of abdominal injury (bowel injury in children). Shoulder belts may cause vascular injuries. Injuries include crush (compression), shear (tearing), and burst (rupture from sudden increase in pressure). Risk of death increases if another vehicle occupant dies. Most frontal collisions result in injuries from impact with the steering wheel, dashboard, windshield, or floorboards. More severe injuries occur at speeds of >25 mph.
Motorcycle crashes	75% of deaths are from head injuries, but injuries to the spine, pelvis, and extremities, including limb loss, are common.
Pedestrian/ Motor vehicle impacts	Often results in Waddell's triad (tibiofibular or femur fracture, trunk injury, and head/face injury). Small children are often run over, and adults are thrown over the car by the impact. Intra-abdominal injuries and pelvic fractures may occur from fender contact with the hips.
Falls	The most common cause of accidental death in geriatric patients is by falling. Anticoagulants increase the risk of injury with falls. The degree of injury depends on patient's weight and fall distance. Injuries are most severe with a fall distance of >20 feet for adults and >10 feet for children. A three-story fall results in 50% mortality; the mortality is almost 100% for five-story falls. Horizontal landings cause fewer injuries (hand, wrist, head/face, and abdominal) than feet-first landings, which often result in fractures of the heel, leg, pelvis, and/or vertebrae.
Sports injuries/ Play	Injuries vary depending on the type of injury but can include head injuries, musculoskeletal injuries, and abdominal injuries. Helmet or knee contact to the flank area may cause kidney injury. The most common injuries are strains, sprains, and knee injuries.
Assaults	Assaults are most common in young males and include facial and head injuries. Severe torso injuries may occur with kicking/stomping. If the patient is intoxicated and has altered consciousness, the patient is treated as having a head injury. Assaults include domestic violence and child abuse, with distinctive patterns of injury.

PENETRATING TRAUMA (BLEEDING)

Gunshot wounds	Solid organs (brain, liver, spleen) often suffer more damage than more elastic tissues (fat, lungs). If a bullet is not deformed after entering the tissue, it tends to tumble (180°), creating a tunnel of injury (permanent cavity) and damage to the surrounding tissue (temporary cavity). If the bullet is deformed, it causes more severe localized tissue damage. Bullets usually have a straight trajectory, but they may be deflected if they strike bone. Shotgun blasts within 15 feet cause more damage than other gunshot wounds, but they are usually less severe at a distance.
Stab wounds	Stab: Includes hand-driven objects (knives, glass shards, ice picks, or pieces of metal/wood). Surface puncture wounds are often small, but their depth varies according to the instrument used, which should be removed surgically. Slash: These are usually long but not deep lacerations. Impalement: This usually results from objects larger than a knife, often from a fall onto an object, but it can include arrows and nails from pneumatic tools.

REVISED TRAUMA SCORE (RTS) AND PRIMARY ASSESSMENT

The **revised trauma score (RTS)** uses the Glasgow Coma Scale (GCS) score, systolic blood pressure (BP), and respiration rate to establish a score for triage (START). Scores may range from 0 to 12. For triage purposes, an RTS of 12 indicates delayed treatment, 11 indicates urgent, and a score of 3 to 10 indicates that immediate treatment is required. Scores less than 3 indicate death. However, the scores are weighted differently, with the GCS score having the greatest weight (RTS = 0.9368 GCS + 0.7326 BP + 0.2908 R), so a reference chart must be used to determine the actual score based on the initial assessment of the patient. **Primary assessment** of trauma patients should include evaluation of the airway, breathing, and circulation (including observing for deviated septum, changes in chest wall motion, fractures, sucking chest wounds, crepitation [of the neck and chest] from air) as well as an assessment of disability with a brief neurological exam (pupils, limb movement) and GSC/RTS. Removing the patient's clothing for examination and logrolling him or her are part of the assessment.

GCS (score)	Systolic BP (score)	Respirations (score)
13-15 (4)	>89 (4)	10-29 (4)
9-12 (3)	76-89 (3)	>29 (3)
6-8 (2)	50-75 (2)	6-9 (2)
4-5 (1)	1-49 (1)	1-5 (1)
3 (0)	0 (0)	0 (0)

TYPES OF BLEEDING

Types of bleeding	Characteristics
Arterial	Bright-red spurting blood that is difficult to control; it lessens as the BP falls.
Venous	Dark-red blood flowing in a steady stream; it, may be copious, but it is easier to control than an arterial bleed.
Capillary	Oozing; it usually clots spontaneously.
Internal	Usually evidenced by increasing signs of shock and/or discolored swollen, painful tissue, guarding, coughing up blood, or rectal bleeding. Long-bone fractures (femur) and pelvic fractures may result in severe blood loss.

PREHOSPITAL

Using standard precautions and PPE as indicated, apply sterile gauze dressing and pressure with the fingertips if it is a small bleed or apply direct hand pressure if it is more copious. As dressings saturate, add new dressings but don't remove the old ones. A tourniquet may be needed if bleeding is uncontrolled. Maintain the patient in the shock position, especially with an arterial bleed or severe blood loss, and keep him or her warm. Avoid giving food or fluids and transport immediately for severe bleeding. Severity relates to the rate of blood loss volume and the age and health of the patient. The blood volume is less with pediatric patients. Moving the injured area, a change in body temperature, medications, and the removal of bandages may impair clotting.

HYPOVOLEMIC SHOCK

Hypovolemic shock occurs when the total circulating volume of fluid decreases, leading to a fall in venous return that in turn causes a decrease in ventricular filling and preload. This results in a decrease in stroke volume and cardiac output. This in turn causes generalized arterial vasoconstriction, increasing afterload (increased systemic vascular resistance), and causing decreased tissue perfusion. Hypovolemic shock is classified according to the degree of fluid loss as follows:

- Class I: <750 mL or ≤15% of total circulating volume (TCV). (This is usually well tolerated.)
- Class II: 750–1500 mL or 15%–30% of TCV. (Tachycardia, anxiety, narrow pulse pressure, and increased respirations.)
- Class III: 1500–2000 mL or 30%–40% of TCV. (Hypotension, pallor, cold, clammy skin, delayed capillary refill, severe tachycardia, and altered mental status.)
- Class IV: >2000 mL or >40% of TCV. (There is severe shock, a weak thready pulse, cyanosis, and death without aggressive resuscitation.)

Prehospital: Control the patient's bleeding; insert two large-bore, short IV catheters; give 250–500 cc warm isotonic boluses (20–30 mL/kg); keep the patient warm; maintain the irway/ventilation/oxygenation to maintain oxygen saturation at 90%–92%; maintain the systolic BP at 70–90 mm Hg; place him or her in the shock position; provide rapid transport.

COMPLICATIONS OF SHOCK

Acute respiratory distress syndrome (ARDS)	Damage to the vascular endothelium and an increase in the permeability of the alveolar–capillary membrane when damage to the lung results from toxic substances; these substances reduce surfactant and cause pulmonary edema as the alveoli fill with blood and protein-rich fluid and then collapse (atelectasis). This decrease in surfactant also leads to decreased lung compliance (sometimes referred to as stiffening). The fluid in the alveoli becomes a medium for infection. Hypoxemia and tachypnea increase as the body tries to compensate to maintain a normal paCO$_2$. Symptoms occur within 72 (usually 24–48) hours of serious injury. Untreated, this condition results in respiratory failure, multiorgan failure, and a mortality rate of 5%–30%. (PEEP is used for ventilation.)
Acute renal failure	The renal tubules are damaged, and the kidneys are unable to filter out the waste products of metabolism.
Multiple-organ failure/dysfunction syndrome (MOFS/MODS)	MOFS/MODS is a progressive deterioration and failure of two or more organ systems with mortality rates of 45%–50% with two organ systems involved and up to 80%–100% if there are three or more systems failing. Trauma patients and those with severe conditions, such as shock, are particularly vulnerable, especially in those >65 years old.

CHEST WOUNDS

Type	Characteristics	Prehospital
Sucking	This is an open pneumothorax in which air sucks into the thoracic cavity, deflating the lung, usually through a penny-size or larger wound. Patients will exhibit respiratory distress, absent breath sounds on the affected side, wound gurgling on inspiration, and bubbling of blood around the wound.	Apply an occlusive dressing with an Asherman Chest Seal dressing or with Vaseline gauze covered with secured (taped on three sides) plastic wrap or aluminum foil and place the patient in position of comfort.
Impalement	This is a penetrating wound with an object impaled into the chest. Symptoms may be similar to those listed above, depending on the site of impalement and the depth. Impalement may cause hemothorax, tension pneumothorax, or pericardial tamponade.	Expose the wound area, and secure the object manually with a bulky dressing. Do not remove the object unless it is necessary for performing chest compressions (CPR). Control the bleeding.

SPECIAL CONSIDERATIONS OF FLUID RESUSCITATION

Special considerations of **fluid resuscitation** include the following:

- Geriatric patients: Underlying hypertension may result in shock with systolic BP >100 mm Hg. Even small amounts of bleeding may lead to shock, especially if the patient has anemia and is less able to tolerate excessive fluids because of underlying anemia or electrolyte imbalances.
- Pediatric patients: Infuse up to 20 mL/kg of warmed isotonic solution, and start a second or third infusion if he or she is nonresponsive to the first infusion. Use continuous infusion for uncontrolled hemorrhage to maintain perfusion en route. It's important to manage temperature control to maintain perfusion. Use an age-specific vital sign chart to monitor vital signs.
- Pregnant patients: Shock results in shunting of maternal blood away from the fetus to the mother's vital organs, so it's critical to maintain the patient's BP as close as possible to normal.

BLUNT CARDIAC TRAUMA

Blunt cardiac trauma most often occurs as the result of motor vehicle accidents, falls, or other blows to the chest, which can result in respiratory distress as well as hypovolemia from rupture of the great vessels of the heart and/or cardiac failure from cardiac tamponade or increasing intrathoracic pressure. The heart is particularly vulnerable to chest trauma, with the right atrium and right ventricle being the most commonly injured because they are anterior to the rest of the heart. *Commotio cordis*, an often-lethal dysrhythmia from a blow to the pericardial area, may occur (most common in young males with sports injuries). Cardiac trauma may be difficult to identify because of other injuries, but if it is suspected, an ECG should be done and any abnormalities (dysrhythmias, ST changes, sinus tachycardia, or heart block) should be noted. Decreased cardiac output and cerebral oxygenation may result in severe agitation with combative behavior. Prehospital: Provide CPR and defibrillation if indicated; manage the patient's airway/ventilation/oxygen supplementation; provide an IV access line with severe injury; monitor changes in the patient's level of consciousness.

FRACTURED RIBS AND FLAIL CHEST

Fractured ribs usually result from severe blunt trauma (motor vehicle accident, physical abuse). Underlying injuries should be expected according to the area of fractures as follows:

- Upper two ribs: Injuries to trachea, bronchi, or great vessels.
- Right-sided ≥ rib 8: Liver trauma.
- Left-sided ≥ rib 8: Spleen trauma.

Pain may be the primary symptom of rib fractures, resulting in shallow breathing. **Flail chest** (more common in adults and adolescents than children) occurs when at least three adjacent ribs are fractured, anteriorly and posteriorly, so that they float free of the rib cage. Variations include the sternum floating with ribs fractured on both sides. With flail chest, the chest wall cannot support changes in intrathoracic pressure, so paradoxical respirations occur with the flail area contracting on inspiration and expanding on expiration. Ventilation decreases. Prehospital: Manage the patient's airway/ventilation/oxygen supplementation (PPV with BVM or intubation), provide cardiac monitoring and supportive care, and observe for signs of tension pneumothorax or hemothorax.

HEMOTHORAX

Hemothorax occurs with bleeding into the pleural space, usually from major vascular injury such as tears in intercostal vessels, lacerations of great vessels, or trauma to lung tissue. It is most common with penetrating wounds. A small bleed may be self-limiting and seal, but a tear in a large vessel can result in massive bleeding, followed quickly by hypovolemic shock from decreased circulating blood. The pressure from the blood may result in the inability of the lung to ventilate and a mediastinal shift. Clots in the chest area may trigger fibrinolysis, which breaks down clots and increases bleeding. Often a hemothorax occurs with a pneumothorax, especially in severe chest trauma. Further symptoms include severe respiratory distress, decreased breath sounds, unequal breath sounds, dullness on auscultation, jugular venous distension, and shock. Prehospital: Manage the patient's airway/ventilation/oxygen supplementation, request assistance for an IV access line and fluid bolus for shock but avoid aggressive fluids because of the risk of hemodilution, provide the patient a position of comfort (the shock position if necessary), and provide rapid transport.

TENSION PNEUMOTHORAX

If not treated promptly, a sucking chest wound (open pneumothorax) may progress to a **tension pneumothorax,** especially if mechanical ventilation is used. A tension pneumothorax occurs when pressure in the pleural space exceeds that of the atmosphere, causing a mediastinal shift (which is usually difficult to assess visually) with displacement of the trachea away from the affected site, putting pressure against the great vessels (decreasing cardiac output) and putting pressure against the heart (resulting in tachycardia). Patients are usually in severe respiratory distress with jugular vein distension, absent breath sounds on the affected side, narrow pulse pressure, pulsus paradoxus, and unequal chest rise. Prehospital: Place an airtight seal or an Asherman Chest Seal over the open wound, manage the patient's airway/ventilation/oxygen supplementation to an oxygen saturation level of ≥94%, provide cardiac monitoring, request assistance for an IV access line, and provide rapid transport. Tension pneumothorax will require needle decompression or insertion of a chest tube (according to protocol).

ABDOMINAL REGIONS OF THE BODY

Abdominal regions include the following:

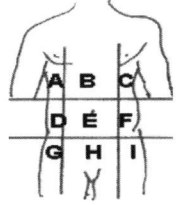

A = Right hypochondriac
B = Epigastric (epi = on, above)
C = Left hypochondriac
D = Right lumbar
E = Umbilical
F = Left lumbar
G = Right iliac
H = Hypogastric (hypo = below, beneath, less than normal)
I = Left iliac

The abdomen may also be divided into four quadrants (sections) with the umbilicus (navel) at the center: right upper quadrant (RUQ), right lower quadrant (RLQ), left upper quadrant (LUQ), and left lower quadrant (LLQ).

PERITONEAL SPACES AND THE ANATOMY OF THE ABDOMINAL AND GENITOURINARY SYSTEMS

The **peritoneum** lines the abdominal cavity. The anterior (front) area is the intraperitoneal space, which contains the stomach, the first part of the duodenum, the small intestines, and part of the large intestines and rectum as well as the liver, bile ducts, spleen, ovaries, part of the pancreas and ureters, and bladder. The posterior (back) retroperitoneal space contains part of the duodenum, the ascending and descending colon and part of the rectum as well as part of the pancreas and ureters, the kidneys, the adrenal glands, the uterus, and the fallopian tubes. The ovaries, uterus, and fallopian tubes comprise the female reproductive system. Solid organs include the liver, spleen, ovaries, uterus, pancreas, kidneys, and adrenals. Hollow organs include the bile ducts, stomach, large and small intestines, fallopian tubes, ureters, and bladder.

ABDOMINAL TRAUMA

Abdominal trauma may result in <u>blunt wounds,</u> which may occur as the result of motor vehicle accidents, motorcycle accidents, pedestrian injuries, sports injuries, falls, blast injuries, and assaults. Blunt injuries comprise crush (compression), shear (tearing), and burst (sudden increased pressure) injuries. Motor vehicle accidents often result in liver injury in the passenger with impact on that side of the vehicle and spleen injury in the driver with impact on the driver's side. Other injuries from blunt trauma include damage to the diaphragm; retroperitoneal hematomas; and intestinal injuries, including perforation. Symptoms of internal injuries include pain, guarding, abdominal distension, discoloration, tenderness on movement, and evidence of lower rib fractures. Some may exhibit rectal bleeding and/or vomiting of blood. Prehospital: Provide airway/ventilation/oxygen supplementation as needed, place in a position of comfort, treat for shock if indicated (especially with suspected internal bleeding), and provide rapid transport for patients in an unstable condition.

Abdominal trauma may result in <u>penetrating wounds,</u> which are almost always related to gunshot wounds (high energy), shotgun wounds (medium energy), or knife wounds (low energy). Gunshot and shotgun wounds tend to cause more extensive damage than stab wounds, especially to the colon, liver, spleen, and diaphragm, and they may have an exit wound. Interior injuries may be extensive because the bullet damages tissues and may ricochet off of bone. Hemorrhage and peritonitis (especially with perforation of the intestines) are common complications. Pain is often more acute with injury to hollow organs than to solid organs, although blood loss may be severe with injury to the liver, spleen, or kidneys, and blood collecting in the retroperitoneal space may not be evident on inspection, palpation, or auscultation. Prehospital: Control external bleeding, manage the patient's airway/ventilation/oxygen supplementation, mobilize the spine if indicated, and apply a pneumatic antishock garment (PASG) if indicated for shock or pelvic fracture (contraindicated with difficulty breathing, pregnancy [second and third trimesters], evisceration, impaled object, and open fractures).

Eviscerations occur with open abdominal wounds, such as opening incisions or traumatic injuries, which allow the internal organs (often the intestines) to protrude externally. Surgical repair is required to reinsert the organs into the abdomen. The patient may go into shock, especially if the evisceration is part of other major injuries (common in trauma cases). Prehospital: Provide supportive care; cover the eviscerated organs with thick sterile gauze dressings moistened with NS, but do not attempt to reinsert the organs; manage the patient's airway/ventilation/oxygen supplementation as needed; and provide rapid transport.

Impalements occur when an object penetrates the abdomen and remains in place and may be associated with multiple internal injuries and bleeding. Prehospital: Do not remove the object, but do expose the abdomen and manually secure the object with bulky dressings, and control any bleeding. Provide supportive care, manage the patient's airway/ventilation/oxygen supplementation as needed, and provide rapid transport.

PNEUMATIC ANTISHOCK GARMENT (PASG)

The **pneumatic antishock garment (PASG)** is indicated for hypovolemic shock and hypotension associated with and stabilization of pelvic and bilateral femur fractures. PASG is contraindicated with respiratory distress, pulmonary edema, pregnancy (second and third trimesters), heart failure, myocardial infarction, stroke, evisceration, abdominal or leg impalement, head injuries, and uncontrolled bleeding above the garment. PASG procedure is as follows:

- Place the garment flat on the patient-transport device/stretcher and transfer the patient onto the garment.
- If the patient is already on the stretcher, place the garment under his or her legs first and then lift the patient's buttocks and slide the garment upward until the upper garment edge is 1 inch below the bottom ribs.
- Secure the legs first and then the abdominal section with the Velcro straps.
- Attach the pump hoses to each leg and the abdominal section at the valves and close the stopcocks.
- Open the stopcock for each leg and abdominal section one at a time, and inflate them one at a time.

- After inflating each section, close the stopcock and check the vital signs. Stop inflating if the systolic BP ≥90 mm Hg. If the systolic BP is still < 90 mm Hg, then proceed to filling the next section until all three are filled.

Traumatic Injuries to Genitalia

Site	Site	Site
Penis	Blunt, penetrating, crushing, or amputating injuries as well as urethral penetration. Pain and bleeding may be severe.	Control external bleeding, do not remove the impaled object. Provide pain management, an ice pack to reduce swelling, and emotional support.
Scrotum	Blunt, penetrating, or crushing injury may result in severe pain and swelling.	As above but do not attempt to relieve scrotal pressure except with ice packs.
Vagina	May have external bruising and tearing (especially with sexual assault) at the vaginal opening. There may be pain, swelling, and bleeding.	Control external bleeding, and provide emotional support, but do not remove impaled objects.
Vulva	May include blunt, penetrating, or crushing injury as well as bite marks (with sexual assault) with pain, swelling, and bleeding.	As above. Report sexual assaults according to protocol.

Orthopedic Trauma

Fractures usually result from trauma (falls, auto accidents), but pathologic fractures can result from minor force to diseased bones (osteoporosis or cancerous lesions). Stress fractures are caused by repetitive trauma (forced marching). Salter-Harris fractures involve the cartilaginous epiphyseal plate near the ends of long bones in children who are growing, and this can impair bone growth. Fracture types are listed as follows:

- Open fractures with soft-tissue injury and a break in the skin overlying the fracture, including puncture wounds from external forces or bone fragments; these can result in osteomyelitis (bone infection).
- Closed fractures involve a broken bone but no break in the skin.

Symptoms include pain, deformity or angulation, swelling, bruising, inability to move the joint or bear weight, grating on movement, and impaired function or circulation. Isolated fractures are usually not life threatening, but pelvic and femur fractures may involve severe blood loss. Prehospital: Cover open wounds with sterile dressings, manually stabilize and immobilize the fracture area but do not replace protruding bones, apply a cold pack, place the patient in a position of comfort.

Subluxation (partial dislocation of a joint) and **luxation** (complete dislocation) can cause neurovascular compromise, which can be permanent if reduction is delayed. This is especially a problem with hip dislocations, which most commonly occur in automobile accidents when the person's knees impact the dashboard. Elbow dislocations often result from athletic injuries and may cause nerve damage. Shoulder dislocations are the most common type and also often result from athletic injuries. They may become chronic. Knee dislocations may result in severe injury to the popliteal artery, and this can lead to amputation, so rapid transport and emergent surgical repair are indicated. Differentiating between fractures and dislocations can be difficult because the symptoms and appearance are often similar. A deformity may not be evident, or it may be obscured by edema, or edema may give the appearance of a deformity. Extensive bruising may occur with all types of injuries, and pain may occur even with minor soft-tissue injuries. Prehospital: Splint and immobilize the area, apply a cold compress, and place the patient in a position of comfort.

Amputations may be partial or complete and result from crush, guillotine (cutting), or avulsion (twisting) injuries. A simple amputation requires no extrication and other injuries or shock are absent, but a complex amputation may involve multiple injuries, shock, and delayed treatment because of extrication. The amputated limb should be treated initially as though it could be reattached, although single digits (except the thumb) and lower limbs are not usually reattached. The part should be irrigated with normal saline (NS) to remove debris; wrapped in NS-moistened gauze; and placed in a sealed plastic bag, which should be immersed in ice water. The body part should not freeze and should not be placed directly on ice. Prehospital: Manage the patient's airway/ventilation/oxygen supplementation; control bleeding by using direct pressure or, if there is severe hemorrhage, by applying a BP cuff proximal to (above) the injury 70 mm Hg greater than the systolic BP for <30 minutes; irrigate the stump with NS if it is dirty; cover the open area with NS-moistened gauze; and elevate the stump.

STRAINS AND SPRAINS

A **strain** is an overstretching of a part of the musculature ("pulled muscle") that causes microscopic tears in the muscle, usually resulting from excess stress or overuse of the muscle. The onset of pain is usually sudden with local tenderness on use of the muscle. A **sprain** is damage to a joint, with a partial rupture of the supporting ligaments and/or tendons, usually caused by wrenching or twisting that may occur with a fall. The rupture can damage blood vessels, resulting in edema, tenderness at the joint, and pain on movement with pain increasing over 2–3 hours after the injury. An avulsion fracture (the bone fragment is pulled away by a ligament) may occur with strain. Prehospital: Immobilize the area for transport, use rest, ice, compression, and elevation (the RICE protocol), and monitor the patient's neurovascular status by checking the pulse, capillary refill, color, and sensation distal to (below) the injury.

PELVIC FRACTURES

Pelvic fractures represent about 3% of total fractures, but they pose a greater risk than most other types of fractures. Pelvic fractures most often result from a motor vehicle accident (50%–60%) in adults and a pedestrian/motor vehicle impact (60%–80%) in children. Pelvic fractures may be accompanied by major injuries to soft tissue and internal organs, especially the bladder, urethra (especially in children and women), and colon. A fracture on one side often results in a fracture on the other side as well. The primary cause of death after a pelvic fracture is hemorrhage with between 50% and 70% of patients with unstable fractures requiring multiple transfusions. Geriatric patients have higher mortality rates than do younger patients. Symptoms include pain and tenderness, bloody urine, rectal bleeding, vaginal bleeding, hematoma over the fracture site, pain on hip motion, and signs of shock (with blood loss). Prehospital: Monitor vital signs for indications of shock, apply PASG or a pelvic wrap device (per protocol) to stabilize and prevent excessive movement, and monitor the patient's airway/ventilation/oxygen supplementation.

TYPES OF FRACTURES

	Transverse: Usually occurs in long bones and is at risk of displacement unless it is splinted to prevent movement. Most often occurs from direct impact, such as sports injuries. May suggest abuse if occurring in small children.
	Comminuted: Usually results from high-impact trauma, such as with motor vehicle accidents, and it is more common in older adults or those with weakened bones. This fracture is very painful and is often accompanied by swelling and muscle spasms.
	Spiral: Common in toddlers who fall on an extended leg, breaking the tibia, but it may also occur with abuse in small children as a result of jerking on or twisting an extremity (usually the arm).
	Displaced: Poses a risk of damage to surrounding tissues, including nerves and blood vessels, and may lead to an open fracture if not properly splinted. Usually the deformity is evident.
	Greenstick: Most common in children whose bones are less hard. It is usually quite painful but without deformity.

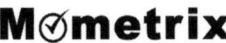

FEMUR/HIP FRACTURES

The femur is the long bone in the thigh. Although any part of the femur may fracture, fractures in the upper femur are common and are generally referred to as hip fractures. **Femur fractures** in young patients usually result from high-impact trauma, such as motor vehicle or pedestrian/motor vehicle accidents, whereas femur fractures in geriatric patients are most often from falls and are associated with osteoporosis. Patients may have many comorbidities and may present with dehydration and blood loss. Mortality rates for hip fractures are high, with 10% during initial treatment and 25% over the next year. Symptoms of femur fractures include pain and deformity at the fracture site and an inability to walk or bear weight. A hematoma may be present. Prehospital: Splint the leg in the position it was found in with a traction splint (Hare Traction Splint/Sager Emergency Traction Splint), flush open fractures with NS to remove debris, and apply an NS-moistened sterile gauze dressing, monitor vital signs and neurovascular status, and assess soft tissue for damage.

PREHOSPITAL MANAGEMENT OF FRACTURES

Fracture	Prehospital
Tibia/Fibula (lower leg)	Manually immobilize during splinting. Splint the joint above and below the fracture(s) (upper thigh to ankle) with a padded rigid long-leg splint or a pneumatic splint, and then secure it to the other leg for additional support.
Shoulder	Apply a sling to the affected side and secure the patient's arm against the body with a swathe to limit movement.
Knee	If the pulse below the fracture is adequate and there is no deformity, splint with the knee straight. If there is deformity, splint the leg in the position it was found. If there is no pulse below the fracture, consult with medical assistance immediately. Never use a traction splint.
Clavicle (upper chest)	Apply a sling to the affected side. (Common in young children who fall with an arm outstretched.)
Humerus (upper arm)	Apply a sling to the affected side and swathe the arm to the body to limit movement.
Radius/Ulna (forearm)	Splint from the elbow to the wrist and secure above and below the fracture. Elevate arm.
Elbow	Apply a sling to the affected side (often results from a fall).

ASSESSMENT OF MUSCULOSKELETAL INJURIES AND THE TYPES OF SPLINTS

Assessment of musculoskeletal injuries should include the following:

- Palpation/Inspection for tissue damage, swelling, deformity, tenderness.
- Comparison with the opposite side if a limb is involved.
- Assessment of neurovascular status (pulse, color, sensation, function) distal to (below) the fracture.
- Assessment of the six P's: <u>pain</u> (site of pain, degree, character), <u>pallor</u> (below the fracture or generalized), <u>paresthesia</u> (impaired sensation below the fracture), distal <u>pulses</u> (intact, weak, absent), <u>paralysis</u> (with or without impaired sensation), and <u>pressure</u> (often associated with swelling and pain).
- Assessment of age and general condition (geriatric patients are more likely to have fractures from minor injuries because of osteoporosis).

If fracture or dislocation is suspected, then the area should be splinted or immobilized for transport. **Types of splints** include rigid (should be padded), nonrigid (moldable), traction, air (pneumatic devices), pillow/blanket, short spine board, and long spine board. Splinting procedures are similar for adults, pediatric patients, and geriatric patients.

COMPARTMENT SYNDROME

Compartment syndrome occurs when muscle perfusion is inadequate because of constriction caused by a cast or tight dressing or because of an increase in the contents of the enclosed compartment of a muscle sheath resulting from edema or hemorrhage, which increases pressure and compression, often related to fractures, crush injuries, burns, rhabdomyolysis, and snakebites. Compartment syndrome most often affects the forearm and leg muscles. Symptoms include severe throbbing pain unrelieved by opiates, numbness and tingling as pressure on the nerves increases, cyanosis and decreased or absent pulse distal to injury, limb paralysis, and edema (with tissue often being rigid). Necrosis and permanent damage may occur within 4 hours if treatment is inadequate or delayed. Prehospital: Remove the constriction (cast, splint, or dressing), elevate the limb, apply an ice compress, provide pain management, and provide rapid transport because the patient may need surgical fasciotomy to relieve the pressure.

OPEN SOFT-TISSUE INJURIES

Injury	Characteristics	Prehospital
Abrasion	Painful superficial scraping of the outermost layer of skin. There is little or no bleeding.	Irrigate with water or NS to remove debris and cover with nonadherent dressing.
Laceration	A cut or break in the skin from impact with a sharp object. Bleeding may vary from mild to severe.	Apply pressure to control the bleeding, irrigate to remove debris if necessary, and cover with a dry sterile gauze dressing.
Puncture	Wound from impact with a sharp pointed object (knife, bullet); it may exhibit little external bleeding but major internal bleeding and soft-tissue damage. An exit wound may be present.	Apply pressure to control any bleeding, manage the patient's airway/ventilation/oxygen supplementation, and provide rapid transport if the patient's condition is unstable.
Impaled object	Penetrating object remains in wound.	Leave the object in place and pad with bulky dressings.
Foreign body in the eye(s)	Patient has pain; tearing; redness; and blurred or impaired vision from dirt, dust, chemicals or other materials in the eye(s).	Cover both eyes loosely (avoiding pressure) to prevent movement. If it is chemical contamination, flush the eye(s) with copious amounts of NS or water.
Avulsions	The skin and underlying soft tissue are torn away, such as with a degloving injury, from any part of the body, although lower extremity injury is the most common. Bleeding may be severe, especially if vessels are torn or exposed.	Flush with sterile water or NS to remove debris if necessary, apply pressure and dressings to control bleeding and protect tissue, apply an ice pack, seal the avulsed skin and tissue in a plastic bag, and place in ice water for possible reimplantation or skin grafts. Return loose flaps to their anatomic positions.
Bites	Extent of the injury varies widely but may involve lacerations, puncture wounds, and avulsions.	As above.
Blast injury	Involves varying degrees of soft-tissue injury and sometimes amputations, fractures, impalements, traumatic brain injuries, ruptured eardrum, pulmonary injury, perforated bowel, and burns.	Manage the patient's airway/ventilation/oxygen supplementation; control bleeding and shock; provide CPR if necessary, supportive care, and rapid transport.

CLOSED SOFT-TISSUE INJURIES

Injury	Characteristics	Prehospital
Contusion	Results from blunt or compressive pressure to a muscle and is a common sports injury. These may include other injuries, such as sprains, strains, fractures, and damage to internal organs. Symptoms include tenderness, pain on movement, and bruising. If bruising is in the shape of an instrument, it usually indicates abuse.	Provide RICE and supportive care.
Hematoma	Collection of blood within the tissue because of damaged blood vessels from injury, underlying fracture, or medications (such as warfarin). These may be small or very large, and patients may lose ≥1 of blood. Symptoms may include pain and swelling.	Provide supportive care for small contusions (which often resolve spontaneously), provide RICE therapy, and monitor for signs of continued bleeding.
Crush injury	External pressure may cause severe internal injuries, such as fractures and organ rupture.	Manage the patient's airway/ventilation/oxygen supplementation and shock as needed, control bleeding, and provide supportive care.

BITE WOUNDS

Injury	Characteristics	Prehospital
Animal bites	Dog bites may cause any type of soft-tissue injury (lacerations, punctures, crush injury, avulsions) depending on the extent of the bite. Cat bites are often puncture bites with a high risk of infection. Pediatric and geriatric patients are most at risk of infection. Children are the most often victims of animal bites.	Check that the scene is safe and the animal is secured, control any bleeding, flush the wound with sterile NS or water, apply dressings, manage the patient's airway/ventilation/oxygen supplementation (especially with bites to the face/throat), and treat shock if needed. Check the rabies status of the animal involved if known. Report the bite according to legal requirements.
Human bites	If the bite is on the genitals, it indicates abuse. Most commonly bites are on the fingers from fist contact with someone's mouth. Human bites are prone to infection, especially if treatment is delayed.	Flush the wound with NS or water, apply a sterile dressing, and provide emotional support for victims of abuse. Document the patient's statement accurately in the event the bite becomes a legal matter.

CLASSIFICATION OF BURNS AND THE RULE OF NINES

Burn injuries may be chemical, electrical, or thermal and are assessed by the area affected, percentage of the body burned, and the depth of the burn, as follows:

- First-degree burns are superficial and affect the epidermis, causing erythema and pain.
- Second-degree burns extend through the dermis (partial thickness), resulting in blistering and sloughing of the epidermis.
- Third-degree burns affect the underlying tissue, including the vasculature, muscles, and nerves (full thickness).

Burns are classified according to the American Burn Association's criteria as follows:

- Minor: <10% body surface area (BSA) or 2% BSA with third-degree burns without serious risk to the face, hands, feet, or perineum.
- Moderate: 10%–20% BSA combined second- and third-degree burns in adults; age <10 years or ≤10% third-degree without serious risk to the face, hands, feet, or perineum.
- Major: 20% BSA; ≥10% third-degree burns; all burns are to the face, hands, feet, or perineum and will result in functional/cosmetic defect; or burns with inhalation or other major trauma.

The rule of nines estimates the BSA burned: Adults—head 9%, trunk (front) 18%, trunk (back) 18%, arm 9%, leg 18%, perineum 1%. Infants/Children—head 18%, trunk (front) 18%, trunk (back) 18%, arm 9%, leg 13.5%, perineum 1%.

Burn Injuries

Burn injuries begin with the skin but can affect all organs and body systems, especially with a major burn. Complications include the following:

- Cardiovascular: Cardiac output may fall by 50% as capillary permeability increases with vasodilation and fluid leaks from the tissues, resulting in hypovolemia and hypothermia. Vasoconstriction occurs as a compensatory mechanism, but it may impair circulation and result in further hypoxia.
- Pulmonary: Injury may result from smoke inhalation or (rarely) aspiration of hot liquid. Pulmonary injury is a leading cause of death from burns and is classified according to the degree of damage as follows:
    - First: Singed eyebrows and nasal hairs with possible soot in airways and slight edema, increasing hypoxia.
    - Second: Stridor, dyspnea, and tachypnea with edema and erythema of the upper airway, including the area of the vocal cords and epiglottis, resulting in severe hypoxia, sometimes with rapid onset.
- Infection: Open wounds are vulnerable to infection.
- Circumferential burns: Swelling beneath eschar can create a tourniquet effect, impairing distal circulation.

Management of Burns

Those with severe burns may develop shock and impairment of all major body systems. If the burning process is ongoing (smoldering clothes, tissue), room-temperature water or NS should be applied to stop the burning and any smoldering clothes or jewelry should be removed, although if the clothing is adhered to the skin, it should be left in place. Facial or airway burns are a major concern, so the airway must be monitored constantly with interventions as necessary. The burned area should be covered with nonadherent clean, dry dressings, and the patient should be kept warm for transport. Children experience greater fluid and heat loss because of their greater body surface area relative to their size, and the AEMT should be alert to the possibility of child abuse. With **chemical burns**, any dry powder should be brushed off and wet chemicals should be flushed with copious amounts of water (by an AEMT wearing gloves and eye protection). With **electrical burns**, internal burns may be more severe than external burns, and the patient is at risk of cardiac arrest.

Dressings and Bandages

Dressing/Bandage	Characteristics
Sterile gauze	4×4 (sponge) or roller/wrapping gauze (Kerlix) that is used to protect skin or pack wounds to control bleeding. Roller gauze may be used to secure other dressings.
Nonadherent dressings	Designed not to stick to open wounds because of their special coating (Teflon, foam, petrolatum, hydrogel). Used on abrasions, burns, and lightly draining wounds.

Dressing/Bandage	Characteristics
Occlusive dressings	These have a waxy coating to make an air- and water-tight seal, but they are not as absorbent as gauze. Used for sucking chest wounds, abdominal eviscerations, and lacerations of the external jugular vein or carotid.
Trauma dressings	Dressings that often include a nonadherent pad, clotting agent embedded in the dressing, and elastic wrap in one piece so that they can be rapidly applied (such as an ACE bandage); these include QuikClot Combat Gauze and Celox Rapid hemostatic gauze. Especially useful to control bleeding and to apply pressure to a wound.
Adhesive, roller bandages	May be elastic or nonelastic, and they are used to secure other dressings and/or apply compression.

HEAD INJURIES

Injury	Characteristics	Prehospital
Head	Open: Bleeding. Closed: Swelling and bruising, may have depression of the skull and underlying injury. Battle's sign (bruising over the mastoid process) and/or raccoon eyes (bruising about the eyes) may indicate a basal skull fracture.	Apply direct pressure to control the bleeding; apply dry, sterile dressings. Monitor the patient's mental status. Be alert for signs of skull fracture.
Scalp	Copious bleeding may occur. May cause shock in infants and young children. Injuries above the ears increase the risk of brain injury.	As above. Manage the patient's airway/ventilation/oxygen supplementation if needed. Rapid transport is required with shock. Avoid closing the patient's mouth with bandages.
Facial	May include soft-tissue damage, facial bone fractures (nasal, orbital), eye injuries, and oral/dental injuries (tooth avulsions, mandibular/maxillary fractures). May have severe swelling, airway compromise, impaired vision, and bloody nose.	Maintain a patent airway, but avoid nasopharyngeal airways; suction as needed; take broken teeth to the hospital; examine the eyes; and control bleeding. Patch both eyes if one or both eyes are injured. Stabilize impaled objects in the eye(s), but remove impaled objects from the cheeks if any bleeding obstructs the patient's airway.

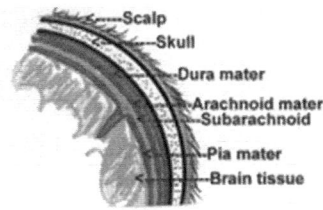

BRAIN AND CERVICAL SPINE INJURIES

Injury	Characteristics	Prehospital
Brain	Direct injury to brain tissue or damage from bleeding inside of the skull may occur, resulting in altered mental status. Cerebrospinal fluid may leak from the nose/ears. Symptoms include the pupils being unequal, nausea and/or vomiting, bradycardia (slow heart rate), increased BP, and irregular breathing. Contusions (bruising) may cause microhemorrhages.	Immobilize the spine; manage the patient's airway/ventilation/oxygen supplementation; provide shock prevention; control bleeding; provide rapid transport.
Spine	Suspect with motor vehicle/pedestrian accidents; falls; hanging; blunt or penetrating trauma to head, neck or torso; diving accidents, and unresponsive trauma patients. May have tenderness in the area; pain on moving; numbness, tingling, or weakness; the inability to feel or move below the injury; difficulty breathing; and incontinence (bowel and/or bladder).	Responsive: Manually stabilize the head and neck in the position found until a cervical collar and backboard are in place. Question the patient's pain, sensations, and ability to move. Unresponsive: Stabilize the head and neck as above; manage the airway, ventilation, and oxygenation; question witnesses; and provide rapid transport.

ANATOMY OF THE BRAIN AND SPINAL CORD

The **brain** is protected by the skull and the meninges, and three layers of lining: the dura mater, arachnoid mater, and the pia mater. Brain tissue is comprised of gray matter (neurons [nerve cells]) and white matter (covered nerve pathways that conduct messages). The main part of the brain is the cerebrum, which is comprised of two hemispheres that contain the frontal parietal, temporal, and occipital lobes. The cerebrum controls higher brain functions, including thoughts, speech, vision, hearing, and actions. The cerebellum lies in the back of the brain below the cerebrum and controls equilibrium and coordination. The brain stem controls involuntary functions, such as respirations, heart rate, temperature control, and nerve transmission. The brain stem is continuous with the **spinal cord**, which is also protected by the meninges and the vertebrae (cervical, thoracic, and lumbar). Cerebrospinal fluid circulates within the subarachnoid space of the brain and the spinal cord.

INTRACRANIAL HEMATOMAS

Type	Characteristics	Prehospital
Epidural	Bleeding between the dura and the skull, pushing the brain downward and inward. The hemorrhage is usually caused by arterial tears, so bleeding is often rapid, leading to severe neurological deficits and respiratory arrest. Patient may be lucid and without symptoms for 2–6 hours after the injury.	Provide supportive care, keep the patient's head elevated to reduce intracranial pressure, note neurological status (movement, strength, mental status, pupils equal and reactive or unequal/fixed), and provide rapid transport.
Subdural	Bleeding between the dura and the arachnoid mater, usually from tears in the cortical veins of the subdural space. It tends to develop more slowly than an epidural hemorrhage. If the bleeding is acute and develops within minutes or hours of injury, then the prognosis is poor. Subacute hematomas that develop more slowly cause varying degrees of injury.	

Type	Characteristics	Prehospital
Intracerebral	Bleeding into the substance of the brain from an artery. Sudden onset; it results in a hemorrhagic stroke with a lack of nutrients and oxygen to parts of the brain. May result from degenerative changes, hypertension, brain tumors, medications, or illicit drugs (crack, cocaine). Symptoms vary depending on the site, but they may include one-sided weakness, paralysis, difficult speaking, severe headache, and altered mental status.	Provide supportive care, keep the patient's head elevated to reduce intracranial pressure, note neurological status (movement, strength, mental status, pupils equal and reactive or unequal/fixed), and provide rapid transport
Subarachnoid	Bleeding in the space between the meninges and brain and into the cerebrospinal fluid, usually resulting from an aneurysm, arteriovenous malformation (AVM), or trauma. This type of hemorrhage compresses the brain tissue. The first presenting symptoms are severe headache, nausea and vomiting, nuchal rigidity, palsy related to cranial nerve compression, retinal hemorrhages, and papilledema.	

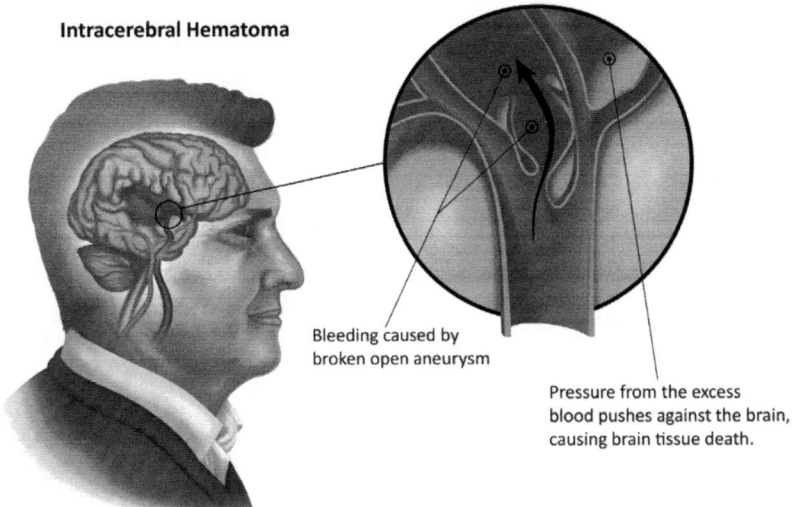

CONCUSSION

Concussion is a brain injury in which structural damage is not apparent but neurological functioning is impaired. Patients may experience a brief loss of consciousness after a head injury and may experience confusion and even bizarre behavior (if the frontal lobe is affected). Other symptoms include severe headache, somnolence, dizziness, lack of coordination, confusion, disorientation, inappropriate emotional response, nausea, and vomiting. Symptoms are usually transient (lasting from minutes to hours), but up to 50% may have recurrent symptoms (such as difficulty concentrating, headaches, and dizziness) for months.

The American Academy of Neurology classifies concussions as follows:

- Grade 1: Transient confusion without loss of consciousness with symptoms resolving in <15 minutes.
- Grade 2: Transient confusion without loss of consciousness with symptoms resolving in >15 minutes.
- Grade 3: Any loss of consciousness of any duration.

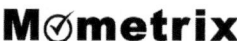

Prehospital: Provide supportive care and reassurance, monitor vital signs and neurological status for signs of increasing intracranial pressure that may indicate more severe injury, and elevate the patient's head.

SIGNS OF INCREASING INTRACRANIAL PRESSURE

Head trauma may result in **increased intracranial pressure** and cerebral edema. Patients often suffer initial hypertension, which increases intracranial pressure and decreases perfusion, and significant swelling, which also interferes with perfusion, causing hypoxia and hypercapnia (increased carbon dioxide), which trigger increased blood flow. This increased volume at a time when injury impairs autoregulation further increases cerebral edema, which, in turn, increases intracranial pressure and results in a further decrease in perfusion with resultant ischemia (impaired circulation). If the pressure continues to rise, the brain may herniate. Symptoms include Cushing's triad: wide pulse pressure, bradycardia, and irregular respirations. Initially: Decreased levels of consciousness, increased BP, and decreased pulse, Cheyne-Stokes (irregular) respirations, pupils reactive. Middle brain stem involvement: Wide pulse pressure, bradycardia, pupils sluggish or nonreactive, hyperventilation. Lower brain stem: Pupil blown on the side of injury, irregular respirations, flaccid response to painful stimulation, and BP and pulse decrease. Prehospital: Elevate the patient's head, manage the patient's airway/ventilation/oxygen supplementation, and provide rapid transport.

NONSPINAL NECK INJURIES AND NASAL FRACTURES

Nonspinal neck injuries may result from blunt trauma or penetrating trauma, and they must be carefully assessed for underlying spinal cord injury. Open wounds may bleed profusely, especially if the carotid artery is breached, resulting in rapid exsanguination and death. The airway may be compromised. Difficulty swallowing indicates esophageal injury, whereas voice changes indicate laryngeal injury. Crackling on palpation indicates air in the tissues. Prehospital: Apply single-digit (gloved) pressure to control bleeding of the carotid artery or jugular veins; apply an occlusive dressing for an injury to large vessels after the bleeding is controlled to prevent air from entering the bloodstream, which is life-threatening; and manage the patient's airway/ventilation/oxygen supplementation (advanced life support may be needed). Rapid or air medical transport may be needed. **Nasal fractures** (40% of facial fractures) may cause persistent bleeding and should be assessed for drainage of the cerebrospinal fluid

and injury of the surrounding structures, including brain injury, skull fracture, and neck and cervical spine injury. Prehospital: Control any bleeding, elevate the patient's head, and manage the airway but do not use nasopharyngeal airways.

FACIAL AND DENTAL INJURIES

Facial injuries may include soft-tissue injuries, fractures, and eye injuries. Facial fractures may result in airway obstruction, pain, swelling, bruising, deformation, and bleeding. Fractures of the maxilla and mandible (the upper and lower jaw) often result in damage to the teeth as well. **Dental fractures,** most commonly of the maxillary teeth, may occur in association with other oral and facial injuries and may be overlooked unless a careful dental examination is carried out. Fractures may range from chipping of the enamel to fracture of the tooth root. **Dental avulsions** are complete displacement of a tooth from its socket. The tooth may be reimplanted if done within 1–2 hours after displacement, although only permanent teeth are reimplanted, not primary teeth, so question the parents of children to determine if an avulsed tooth is permanent. Prehospital: Manage the patient's airway/ventilation/oxygen supplementation as needed, elevate the patient's head, and place the avulsed tooth in NS for transport.

Unstable facial fractures are those of the midface, usually from blunt facial trauma and are often associated with other trauma because of the degree of force involved. Categories include the following:

- Le Fort I (low downward force): The hard palate and lower maxilla are separated from the rest of skull.
- Le Fort II (low or mid-maxilla force): The nasal bones and lower maxilla are separated from the facial skull and other cranial bones.
- Le Fort III (force to the bridge of the nose or the upper maxilla): The entire midface is separated from the cranium.

Symptoms may include malocclusion, open bite, apparent lengthening of the face, clear nasal discharge (cerebrospinal fluid), periorbital ecchymosis, pain, swelling, and epistaxis (nosebleed), vision disturbances, airway compromise. Prehospital: Suction if necessary, manage the patient's airway/ventilation/oxygen supplementation (usually with intubation; avoid a nasopharyngeal airway), control any bleeding, elevate the patient's head. (Cricothyroidotomy may be necessary if the airway is obstructed.) Patch both eyes if one or both are injured. Stabilize an impaled object in the eye, but remove an impaled object in the cheek; apply dry sterile dressings, but do not cover the mouth; provide rapid transport.

MANDIBULAR FRACTURES, LARYNGOTRACHEAL INJURIES, AND NON-CNS-ASSOCIATED SPINAL TRAUMA

Mandibular fractures are most common in males 21 to 30 and result from a blow to the jaw from an assault, motor vehicle accident, or gunshot wound and are often associated with other injuries, such as head injury or midface fractures. Symptoms include malocclusion of teeth, pain, point tenderness, and ecchymosis of the floor of the mouth. Prehospital: Manage the patient's airway/ventilation/oxygen supplementation (avoid the nasal airway), use an ice pack to reduce edema, elevate the patient's head, and monitor him or her closely.

Laryngotracheal injuries result from direct trauma and may result in swelling and hemorrhage. Symptoms include swelling, changes in voice, hemoptysis, subcutaneous emphysema (from open wounds), and structural irregularities. The patient must be assessed for associated injuries. Prehospital: Manage the patient's airway/ventilation/oxygen supplementation because airway obstruction is common, elevate the patient's head, and provide supportive care. The patient may require a surgical airway.

With **non-CNS-associated spinal trauma,** patients complain of pain and point tenderness, but neurological findings are intact. Prehospital: Provide sitting or standing spinal mobilization and supportive care; manage the patient's airway/ventilation/oxygen supplementation as needed.

ANATOMY AND PHYSIOLOGY OF THE EYE AND EYE CONDITIONS

The **eyes** fit into sockets (orbits) in the skull. The eyelid and sclera are lined with conjunctiva (clear tissue). The outer layer of the eye is the cornea, which focuses light. The pupil (at the center) dilates or constricts to control light coming into the eye. The iris (the colored part) adjusts the size of the pupil. The lens is behind the pupil and allows the eyes to focus. The vitreous humor is the gel-like substance in the middle of the globe. The retina at the back of the eye transmits visual images to the brain. The sclera (white part) contains blood vessels and protects the eye.

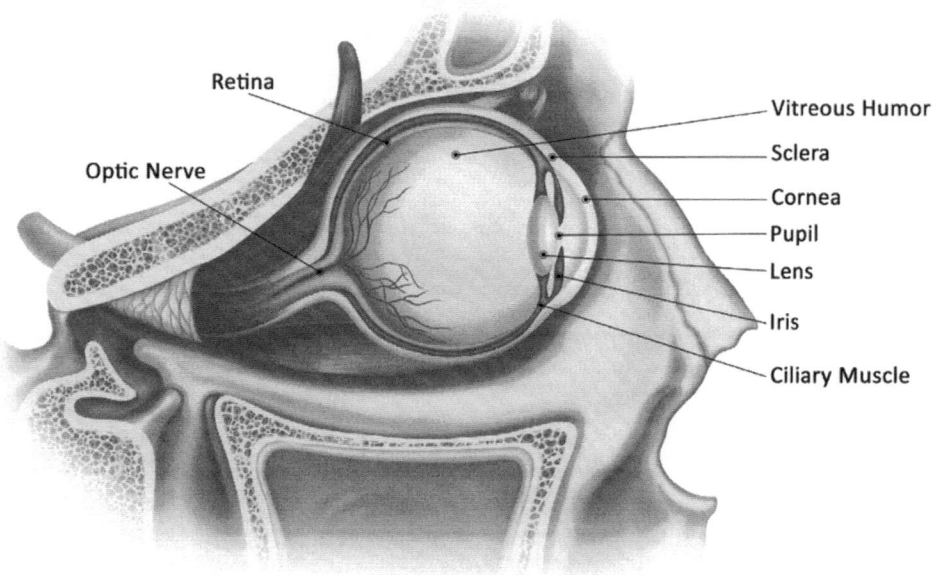

Eye Condition	Characteristics	Prehospital
Burns	Chemical/fire: Pain, tearing, difficulty opening the affected eye.	Irrigate with NS or sterile water for 20–30 minutes.
Corneal abrasion (scratch)/ Foreign body	Often associated with a failure to use safety glasses or wearing contact lenses. A foreign body may remain in the eye(s). Symptoms: Blurred vision, pain, tearing, photophobia, and squinting (muscle spasms).	As above. Do not attempt to remove a foreign body; patch both eyes to prevent movement.

ORBITAL FRACTURES AND PERFORATED TYMPANIC MEMBRANE

Orbital fractures most often occur with blunt force against the globe causing a rupture through the floor of the orbital bone or a direct blow to the orbital rim, often related to an assault or sports injury. Injuries are most common in adolescents and young adults. Patients may be essentially asymptomatic, or they may exhibit ecchymosis and edema of the eyelid, infraorbital anesthesia from pressure or damage to the infraorbital nerve, decreased sensation of the cheek and upper gum on the injured side, diplopia (double vision), and enophthalmos (sunken globe). Prehospital: Patch both eyes to prevent movement, provide supportive care, and use an ice compress to reduce edema.

A **ruptured tympanic membrane** may result from pressure (diving, waterskiing), a direct blow to the ear, explosions, and a foreign object in the ear. Symptoms may include pain, hemorrhagic otorrhea (bloody drainage), and hearing impairment. Prehospital: Provide supportive care.

SKULL FRACTURES

The skull is divided into eight cranial bones: one frontal bone (over the frontal lobe), two parietal bones (over the parietal lobes), two temporal bones (over the temporal lobes), one occipital bone (over the occipital lobe and cerebellum), one sphenoid bone (it forms part of the eye orbit), and one ethmoid bone (it separates the nasal cavity from the brain). **Skull fractures** include the following:

- Basilar: Occurs in the bones at the base of the brain and can cause severe brain stem damage.
- Comminuted: The skull fractures into small pieces.
- Compound: A surface laceration extends to a skull fracture, which may be overlooked because of heavy bleeding.
- Depressed: May be open and is often comminuted. Pieces of the skull are depressed inward on the brain tissue, often producing dural tears and underlying brain trauma.
- Linear/hairline: A skull fracture forms a thin line without any splintering, usually without any underlying injury.
- Diastatic: Affects children younger than 3 years old, widening the skull sutures.

SPINAL INJURIES AND SPINAL CORD INJURIES

Spinal injuries of the vertebrae include fractures, dislocations, open wounds, and flexion and extension injuries. Because the spinal cord lies within the vertebral column, injury to the vertebrae may cause **spinal cord injuries** and disrupt transmissions in nerves that connect the body and the brain. Spinal cord injuries may affect only a few nerves, or they may completely transect the spinal cord, resulting in permanent paralysis below the site of injury. Spinal cord injuries should be suspected with head trauma, penetrating trauma, direct blunt trauma, falls, diving injuries, motor vehicle accidents, rapid deceleration accidents, and multisystem trauma. Assessment includes evaluating extremity movement, respiration control, sensation, pain/tenderness, and vital signs. Prehospital: Logroll the patient to examine his or her back, immobilize the patient (seated or standing), apply a rigid cervical collar, lift and move him or her with care, and provide rapid transport. Elevate the torso of children 2–3 cm with padding so that the head is in a neutral position if using an adult immobilization device. Immobilize infants in their car seats, padding all the voids.

BRAIN INJURIES, THE COUP/CONTRECOUP PATTERN, AND POSTURING

Primary brain injuries are those that result from the original trauma and include direct damage to brain tissue, such as may occur with a gunshot wound. **Secondary brain injuries** result from the effects of the primary injury, such as increasing intracranial pressure, ischemia (most common), hemorrhage, edema, and brain herniation. **Coup/Contrecoup** injuries are common in motor vehicle accidents and shaken baby syndrome. With acceleration/deceleration and contact injuries where the head hits a fixed object (such as a windshield) and snaps back from the impact, *coup* (on the side of impact) and contrecoup (on the opposite side) contusions may both occur. **Decerebrate (extension) posturing** (with the body stiff, legs straight, feet extended, arms straight, and the head/neck arched back) is associated with severe midbrain damage. **Decorticate (flexion) posturing** (with the body stiff, legs straight, and hands clenched on the chest) is associated with damage to the pathway connecting the brain and spinal cord and may include damage to the cerebral cortex, white matter, or basal ganglia.

PREGNANCY TRAUMA

The mother and fetus are each considered to be patients. Trauma is the cause of 46% of maternal deaths, and blunt trauma is the cause of up to 38% of fetal deaths. Pregnant patients are susceptible to falls (especially in the third trimester when the mother's center of gravity shifts) and domestic abuse (which may include blunt trauma and penetrating trauma from knife or gunshot wounds). However, most trauma in pregnant women occurs as the result of motor vehicle accidents. Pregnant women have an increased blood volume and heart rate, impaired venous return if in a supine (flat) position in the third trimester, and increased risk of vomiting and aspiration. Hypovolemia/shock reduces the amount of oxygen to the fetus, resulting in fetal stress. Vaginal bleeding may occur. Prehospital: Have suction available, monitor the patient's airway/ventilation/oxygen supplementation, and provide 100% oxygen per nonrebreather mask and ventilation assistance if needed (especially with symptoms of shock), transport on the left side (tilt the immobilization board if necessary), and provide rapid transport.

Pediatric Trauma

Note the pediatric assessment triangle (appearance, work of breathing, and circulation). Respiration rates vary with age, but the use of accessory muscles and sternal retraction indicate respiratory distress. Assess the brachial pulse in infants—a slow pulse indicates hypoxia. Trauma is the leading cause of death in pediatric patients, and hypoventilation is the leading cause of cardiac arrest. BP values are not reliable for small children, who may have normal BP in compensated shock. Shaken baby syndrome should be considered with pediatric trauma; it is believed to be the result of vigorous shaking of an infant, causing acute subdural hematoma (brain hemorrhage) and retinal (eye) hemorrhages. It is believed that the shaking of the brain causes coup (front) and contrecoup (back) damage as well as damaging the vessels and nerves with resultant cerebral edema (swelling). Prehospital: Manage hypovolemia/shock, prevent hypothermia, and manage the patient's airway/ventilation/oxygen supplementation as needed. Ventilate if the patient is bradycardic. BVM ventilation is usually the best ventilation method for children.

Geriatric Trauma

These patients are more susceptible to trauma because of aging processes, and they may be less able to maintain normal vital signs during hemorrhage. About 80% of patients older than age 65 have one chronic illness, and 50% have two. Polypharmacy is common, and medications may affect vital signs and blood clotting. Response times may be slower than normal Falls are the most common cause of injury in geriatric patients. Elder abuse should be suspected if patients have repeated injuries. Scalding is the most common burn injury and is often deeper because of thinning skin. The risk of cerebral bleeding with trauma is increased because of brain shrinkage. The cough reflex may be lessened. Fractures are common because of osteoporosis, especially hip fractures. Prehospital: Splint fractures, monitor the patient's airway/ventilation/oxygen supplementation, monitor oxygenation with pulse oximetry, suction if necessary, and check the mouth for dentures (which may obstruct the airway). Note: Spinal curvature may require padding of the spinal board.

Trauma in Cognitively Impaired Patients

Disorders may include Alzheimer's or other forms of dementia, traumatic brain injuries, strokes, Down's syndrome, and autistic spectrum disorders, so patients may be of all ages. Patients may be more at risk of trauma, and assessment and history taking may be difficult. Perceptions of pain may be altered, and psychological reactions may vary. Patients who are cognitively impaired are often more vulnerable to physical, sexual, and psychological abuse and may be unable to or afraid to report abuse. Patients may have an exaggerated response to pain or injury and may be very frightened and agitated or withdrawn, so the extent of the injury may be difficult to determine. Prehospital: Remain supportive, reassure the patient, avoid any use of medical jargon, use simple statements (asking one question at a time), use yes/no questions, obtain information from the caregiver if necessary, and treat as indicated by the patient's condition.

Generalized Hypothermia

Generalized hypothermia occurs when the body temperature falls to below-normal levels.

- Mild: 32°C–35°C (89.6°F–95°F).
- Moderate: 28°C–32°C (82.4 °F–95°F).
- Severe: <32°C (<82.4°F).

Contributing factors include wet and cold environments, wind, age (geriatric/pediatric), medical conditions, substance abuse (alcohol, drugs), and poison. Up to 50% of trauma patients with severe injuries become hypothermic because of exposure, blood loss, shock, and standard procedures (such as administration of cold fluids and clothing removal). Indications of hypothermia include cold skin, shivering, decreased mental status (confusion, memory loss, lethargy, dizziness, mood changes, impaired judgment, difficulty speaking), decreased sensation of touch, decreased motor function (muscle rigidity, stiff posture, muscle/joint stiffness), and bradycardia (slow pulse). Prehospital: Remove the patient from the cold environment, remove any wet clothing, wrap in warm blankets, begin CPR if no pulse is obtained after 30–45 seconds of assessment, and use an AED if it indicates the need to defibrillate.

HEAT-RELATED ILLNESSES

Condition	Characteristics	Prehospital
Heat stress	Increased temperature causes dehydration. Symptoms may include swelling of the hands and feet, flushing, itching, sunburn, dizziness, muscle cramps, and hyperventilation. The patient's temperature is normal.	Remove the patient from heat, give fluids to rehydrate, and give oxygen with a nonrebreather mask.
Heat exhaustion	Dehydration results in sodium depletion. Symptoms may include flu-like symptoms, headache, dizziness, fainting, nausea, vomiting, weakness, muscle cramping, rapid pulse, diaphoresis, and cold clammy skin. The patient's temperature is usually <106°F (41°C), and it may be normal.	Remove the patient from heat; use evaporative cooling techniques such as ice packs to the axilla, groin, and neck; and rehydrate (one-half glass of fluid every 15 to 20 minutes). Give oxygen as above.
Heat stroke	There are two types, which may progress to multiorgan dysfunction syndrome with liver and kidney failure, and death. <u>Exertional:</u> Sudden onset after exertion. The patient's temperature varies because he or she is still sweating; there is diaphoresis, syncope, and loss of consciousness. <u>Nonexertional:</u> Sudden onset after heat exposure. The temperature is usually >106°F (41°C) rectally or >103°F (39.4°C) orally. There can be mild irritability, decorticate posturing, seizures, coma, and tachycardia.	Remove the patient from heat, apply evaporative cooling and ice packs as above, provide airway/ventilation/oxygenation support as needed, and provide rapid transport.

FROSTBITE/FREEZING

Frostbite is tissue damage from **freezing**, most often affecting the nose, ears, and distal extremities (hands/feet). The affected part feels numb and aches or throbs, becoming hard and insensate as the tissue freezes, resulting in circulatory impairment, necrosis of tissue, and gangrene. Degrees of frostbite/freezing are as follows:

1. Partial freezing with redness and mild swelling, stinging, burning, and throbbing pain.
2. Full-thickness freezing with increased swelling in 3–4 hours and clear blisters in 6–24 hours; sloughing of skin with eschar formation, numbness, and then aching and throbbing pain.
3. Full-thickness freezing into the subdermal tissue with cyanosis, hemorrhagic blisters, skin necrosis, a "wooden" feeling, severe burning, throbbing, and shooting pains.
4. Freezing extends into the subcutaneous tissue (muscles, tendons, and bones) with a mottled appearance, nonblanching cyanosis, and eventually deep black eschar.

Prehospital: Remove the patient from the cold environment, handling him or her with care; remove wet clothing; cover the patient with a blanket; remove jewelry; manually stabilize the affected area; and transport rapidly. Do NOT break blisters, rub or massage the area, apply heat, rewarm if the area may refreeze, allow the patient to walk, or give him or her anything by mouth.

DECOMPRESSION SICKNESS

Decompression sickness (dysbarism) occurs when a diver ascends too quickly and the body is unable to compensate for the pressure change. Because the pressure reduces too rapidly, dissolved gases in the blood, such as helium and nitrogen, form bubbles. These bubbles interfere with blood flow and can cause gas emboli, which can obstruct blood vessels and damage the alveoli in the lung. The gas emboli can affect all tissues, with symptoms ranging from mild to severe to complete neurological and cardiovascular collapse. Typical mild to moderate symptoms include joint pain, numbness, tremors, amnesia, difficulty breathing, itch, tinnitus, vertigo, and localized swelling. Severe symptoms include pneumothorax, loss of consciousness, seizures, weakness, or paralysis of extremities. Onset of mild symptoms is gradual with more than 40% having symptoms within one hour, but the onset of severe symptoms may occur within minutes of surfacing. Prehospital: Rapid transport for recompression therapy is critical to survival (especially in severe cases); manage the patient's airway/ventilation/oxygen supplementation with 100% oxygen through a nonrebreather mask. Air transport must be below 1000 feet in altitude.

SUBMERSION/DROWNING

Submersion may cause aspiration (wet drowning) or trigger severe laryngospasm (dry drowning), although some people will be pulled from the water still breathing. **Drowning** is the leading cause of death in children younger than age 5, and it is the second leading cause of death in children younger than age 15. Most infant submersions are in bathtubs and result from intentional injury or lack of supervision. Adolescent/Adult submersions are often related to drugs, alcohol, or risk-taking behaviors. Submersion asphyxiation can cause profound damage to multiple organ systems, including the brain, heart, and lungs, from lack of oxygen and aspiration. Hypothermia related to near drowning has some protective effect because blood is shunted to the brain and heart. Indications of submersion include coughing, vomiting, difficulty breathing, and respiratory and cardiac arrest. Prehospital: Initiate CPR if the patient is in arrest, manage the patient's airway/ventilation/oxygen supplementation with 100% oxygen (the patient may need intubation), place the patient in the recovery position if he or she is unconscious or vomiting, provide suction as needed, and provide rapid transport.

ELECTRICAL INJURIES

Low-voltage **electrical contact** most often causes a localized burn (first to third degree) to the hand or mouth (toddlers) with various degrees of tissue damage, although mouth contact may also result in cardiac or respiratory arrest. High-voltage electrical contact results in an entry and an exit wound with internal damage occurring between these wounds. Electrical current takes the shortest route to leave the body (flowing along blood vessels and nerves), so if the current passes from hand to hand, damage is usually more severe than if it passes from a hand to a foot. Severe injury may result in damage to bones, compartment syndrome, organ failure, and cardiac arrest from asystole or ventricular fibrillation. Vessels may be mildly or severely damaged. Abdominal organs may be damaged. Neurological damage with unconsciousness is common, especially if the current passes through the head. Peripheral nerve damage is also common, and damage to the spinal cord may occur. Prehospital: Manage the patient's airway/ventilation/oxygen supplementation, provide CPR/defibrillation as needed, and provide rapid transport (with the head elevated if it was involved).

LIGHTNING INJURIES

Lightning injuries may occur with a direct strike (≤5%), side splash from a strike nearby, contact voltage when touching an item that has been struck, ground current (from a more distant strike), and blunt trauma from being too close to a strike (which often results in the patient being thrown). Symptoms may vary, but they can include external burns (Lichtenberg figures) in a fernlike pattern, acute pain, fixed and dilated pupils (temporary), eye injuries, confusion, headache, hearing loss, perforated eardrum, hypotension, paralysis/paresis, spinal cord injury, altered mental status, brain injury, fractures, and cardiac arrest. Patients may be responsive initially but lapse into unconsciousness as cerebral edema increases, resulting in secondary respiratory and/or cardiac arrest. Burns are usually mild because of the brief contact. Prehospital: Manage the patient's airway/ventilation/oxygen supplementation, provide CPR/defibrillation as needed, and provide rapid transport (with the head elevated).

INSECT BITES

Injury	Characteristics	Prehospital
Fire ants	Hives and blistering with severe itching, redness, pain, and burning. Some patients may develop systemic reactions and anaphylaxis.	Provide supportive care and cold compresses. Use the anaphylaxis protocol if necessary.

Injury	Characteristics	Prehospital
Wasps/bees	Pain, itching, redness, and swelling (most common). Severe allergic (hives) and/or anaphylactic (life-threatening) reactions.	Wipe the area with gauze or scrape it with a sharp instrument to remove the stinger, wash with soap and water, apply ice, and elevate. Use the anaphylaxis protocol if necessary.
Scorpions	May cause local (burning, itching, pain, and redness) or severe neurologic and/or other systemic reaction, such as paresthesia, stroke, hypertension, tachycardia, respiratory distress, priapism, hemorrhage, nausea, and vomiting. Pregnant women may miscarry.	Immobilize the affected part below the level of the heart, apply cool compresses (the first 2 hours), monitor the patient's airway/ventilation/oxygen supplementation, and provide rapid transport.
Ticks	Pain may occur at the bite site. Ticks may carry numerous infections, including Lyme disease, so follow-up is essential.	Grasp the tick near the skin with tweezers and pull with steady upward pressure, disinfect the site, and save the tick in a plastic bag.

SPIDER BITES

Injury	Characteristics	Prehospital
Black widow	Initially there are two faint fang marks with a pale area surrounded by a red-blue ring. Muscle cramps, pain radiating to the upper chest (arm bites) or abdomen (leg bites) and weakness within 2 hours increasing to generalized pain, headache, itching chills, nausea, vomiting, dyspnea, hypertension, cardiac abnormalities, shock, and coma.	Provide supportive care and analgesia. Take the spider in a sealed plastic bag to the receiving facility.
Brown recluse	Red, swollen bite site with severe pain and itching; "red, white, and blue" sign—a pale center with a central blister and reddish-blue peripheral discoloration with the blister becoming ischemic and necrotic—leaving an open ulcerated area that covers with black eschar and may expand in size. The following systemic reactions may occur within 6–12 hours in some patients: fever, vomiting, jaundice, hypotension, change in mental status, hemolytic anemia, disseminated intravascular coagulation, renal failure, seizures, coma, and death.	

SNAKEBITES

Pit vipers include rattlesnakes, copperheads, and cottonmouths. They have erectile fangs that fold until they are aroused; their venom is primarily hemotoxic and cytotoxic, but it may also have neurotoxic properties (affecting the blood, cells, and nerves at the bite site and systemically). Symptoms vary depending on the amount of venom that is injected (many bites are dry).

- Wounds usually show one or two fang marks.
- Swelling may begin immediately, or it may be delayed for up to 6 hours.
- Pain may be severe.
- There may be a wide range of symptoms, including hypotension and impairment of blood clotting that can lead to excessive blood loss, depending upon the type and amount of venom.
- Progressive weakness, vision problems, nausea and vomiting, altered consciousness, and seizures are expected.

Prehospital: Note the time elapsed from the time of the bite to the time of transport, reassure the patient, immobilize the extremity, cleanse the wound with soap and water, apply an ice pack to slow venous return and reduce swelling, transport immediately for further treatment such as with antivenom, and mark the extent of swelling on the skin every 15 minutes.

MULTISYSTEM TRAUMA

Multisystem trauma (common) involves injury to more than one major system. Care includes the following points:

- Ensure the safety of the patient and all rescue personnel, and determine the need for additional resources.
- Consider the mechanism of injury and identify and manage life-threatening conditions.
- Manage the patient's airway/ventilation/oxygen supplementation (high concentration) as well as the necessary spinal immobilization with him or her in a lying/sitting position, and make positioning decisions.
- Control hemorrhage and provide shock therapy and maintain body temperature.
- Splint musculoskeletal injuries.
- Suspect additional injuries.
- Prioritize interventions and continue care en route rather than delaying transport.
- Evaluate the patient's condition by the injuries sustained (bleeding, difficulty breathing, lack of pulse) rather than by the patient's response (screaming, yelling).
- Complete the primary and secondary assessments, and obtain a medical history.
- Platinum ten—the first 10 minutes on the scene in which the patient should be extricated and stabilization efforts should be started.
- Golden hour—the first 60 minutes during which the patient should be stabilized and transported to the receiving facility.
- Notify the receiving facility so resources are prepared.

BLAST INJURIES

Blast injuries may result from high-order explosives (TNT, nitroglycerin) or low-order explosives (pipe bombs, Molotov cocktails). Enclosed explosions usually cause more injury than do open-air blasts. Blast waves occur only with high-order explosives and result from high-pressure impulses. Blast wind may occur with either type of explosives and involves superheated air. Ground shock may cause further injury. Immediate death may occur. Injuries may include the following:

Type	Characteristics	Prehospital
Primary	Blast wave injury affects gas-filled organs/structures: lungs, eardrum, abdomen, eyes, and brain (20% of victims).	Be alert for a second explosive device or a device on a victim (who may be a perpetrator). Carry out rapid triage. Control any bleeding/manage shock. Manage the patient's airway/ventilation/ oxygen supplementation. Provide CPR if necessary. Splint musculoskeletal injuries. Provide rapid transport.
Secondary	Penetrating injuries from flying shrapnel affecting any part of the body along with abrasions, contusions, and lacerations. (Secondary injury is the most common cause of death.)	
Tertiary	Injuries from being thrown by blast wind: fractures, spinal and brain injuries, and traumatic amputations.	
Quaternary	Other injuries and complications, such as difficulty breathing because of smoke inhalation, burns, and crush injuries.	

Special Patient Populations

Premonitory Signs of Labor

Lightening	As the fetal head engages and moves toward the birth canal, the fundal pressure on the diaphragm lessens, so the mother can breathe more easily, but pressure in the pelvic area increases, causing urinary frequency. The lower abdomen may protrude more than previously. Increased circulatory impairment may cause venous stasis and ankle swelling as well as increased vaginal secretions as the vaginal mucous membranes become congested. Pressure on the nerves may result in leg cramps or pelvic and leg pain.
Braxton Hicks (BH)	BH contractions are short in duration, occur at irregular intervals in the lower abdomen, and do not change the cervix. They are often relieved by activity or mild analgesia. The intensity and frequency of BH contractions often increase immediately prior to the onset of true labor.
Cervical changes	The cervix ripens (softens) to allow for effacement (thinning) and dilation.
Bloody show	A mucous plug from pooled secretions forms at the opening of the cervical canal during pregnancy, and when the cervix begins to efface, this mucous plug is expelled, exposing capillary vessels that bleed. The bloody show typically appears as pink mucus. Bloody show usually occurs within 24 to 48 hours of the onset of labor.
Ruptured membranes	Rupture of the membranes occurs in about 12% of women prior to the onset of labor, which usually then occurs within 24 hours. Before rupture, the membranes typically bulge through the dilating cervix; fluid comes in a gush, although it may come in smaller spurts in some cases. If the membranes rupture before engagement of the fetal head, the umbilical cord may prolapse with the fluid, increasing risk to the fetus, so mothers should always seek medical attention after rupture. If the mother is at term and labor does not start within 24 hours of rupture, labor may be induced.

Stages of Labor

First	Latent phase: The cervix begins to dilate; contractions are mild to moderate and occur every 3–30 minutes and are of short duration. Active phase: The cervix is dilated to 4–7 cm; contractions are every 1–5 minutes, lasting 20–40 seconds. Pain is increased. Transitional phase: The cervix is fully dilated (8–10 cm); contractions come every 1.5–2 minutes, lasting 60–90 seconds. There is increased pain, hyperventilation, crying, moaning, vomiting, and rectal pressure.
Second	From fully dilated cervix to delivery with contractions as in the transitional phase. The perineum begins to bulge, and the fetal head crowns as the mother begins to bear down and birth is imminent. Pressure on the rectum and anus may cause stool to be expelled. Birth occurs head first if it is a normal delivery, feet first if it is a breech delivery.
Third	Delivery of the placenta should occur 5–30 minutes after birth. Retained placenta occurs if more than 30 minutes elapse.
Fourth	The period of 1–4 hours after birth, which involves 250–400 mL blood loss, moderate hypotension (low BP), and tachycardia (rapid pulse).

ORGANS OF PREGNANCY AND VAGINAL BLEEDING

Organs of pregnancy include the uterus (womb). The placenta is attached to the walls of the uterus; it includes the umbilical cord, which provides blood, nutrients, and oxygen to the fetus. The fetus is inside an amniotic sac, which contains amniotic fluid that cushions the fetus. The opening to the uterus is the cervix, which thins and dilates for delivery. The vagina provides the birth canal.

Vaginal bleeding during the first trimester of pregnancy may indicate spontaneous abortion, ectopic pregnancy, or infection, although light occasional spotting may be normal. All vaginal bleeding during pregnancy should be assessed by a physician, and a large amount of bleeding may indicate a medical emergency. "Bloody show" near term may indicate that delivery is near. Prehospital: Use standard precautions, and position the patient on her left side. Place a sanitary pad over the vaginal opening, and save any soaked pads in a plastic bag so the physician can estimate the amount of blood loss. Manage the patient's airway/ventilation/oxygen supplementation, and provide emotional support. Provide an IV access line and fluids if indicated.

SPONTANEOUS AND ELECTIVE ABORTION AND ECTOPIC PREGNANCY

Spontaneous abortion: Unplanned loss of pregnancy at or before 20 weeks. May result from trauma, fetal abnormality, or another cause. Indications include vaginal bleeding (mild to severe) and contractions. The patient may be very emotionally upset. Prehospital: Use the term "miscarriage" rather than "abortion," which has negative connotations for many; gather any products of conception in a plastic bag to take to the hospital; provide supportive care; place a sanitary pad over the vagina; and provide reassurance and emotional support.

Elective abortion: Planned loss of pregnancy at or before 20 weeks per surgical procedure or abortion pills (during the first 10 weeks). Patients may develop bleeding after surgery or as the fetus is expelled. Prehospital: Gather any products of conception in a plastic bag to take to the hospital, provide supportive are, place a sanitary pad over the vagina, and provide reassurance and emotional support.

Ectopic pregnancy: Pregnancy in which the egg fertilizes and attaches outside of the uterus (usually in the fallopian tubes), resulting in abdominal pain, absent menstrual periods, and vaginal bleeding. Prehospital: As above.

DELIVERY OF A NEWBORN

If the fetal head is obvious at the vaginal opening (crowning), **delivery** is imminent. Steps to delivery include the following:

- Wash hands and don PPE for standard precautions and obtain an OB kit and supplies.
- Position the patient on her back with hips elevated, knees bent, and legs apart.
- Position one person at the mother's head for support if possible while the other supports the baby's head during delivery.
- Provide oxygen to the mother.
- If the umbilical cord is around the baby's neck, attempt to slip it over the infant's head.
- Make note of the time of delivery.
- Lower the infant's head to facilitate drainage of fluids, and keep the mouth and nose suctioned with a bulb syringe.
- Clamp the cord or cut it if sterile equipment is available.
- Monitor the infant's airway, breathing, and circulation with the baby at the level of the birth canal.
- Monitor delivery of the placenta (afterbirth).
- If mother and infant are stable, allow the infant to nurse.
- Place a sanitary pad over the vaginal opening to contain any bleeding. Observe for hemorrhage.
- Massage the uterus in a circular motion to prevent excessive bleeding.

COMPLICATIONS OF PREGNANCY AND LABOR

Complication	Characteristic	Prehospital
Preterm labor	Labor between weeks 20 and 37; presents a risk to the fetus.	Provide supportive care. Manage the patient's airway/ventilation/oxygen supplementation (100%). Transport rapidly if there is severe bleeding or a risk of imminent preterm delivery.
Premature rupture of membranes	Membranes rupture before the onset of labor; this may lead to preterm labor and risk to the fetus.	
Substance abuse	May result in damage to the fetus and preterm labor. Many drugs restrict blood flow to the fetus, resulting in growth restriction and low oxygen. Some drugs, such as cocaine, affect the fetal nervous system. Sudden withdrawal of opiates may trigger preterm labor. Alcohol may result in fetal alcohol syndrome, characterized by facial abnormalities, growth restriction, and neurological defects.	
Placental abruption	The placenta prematurely detaches, partially or completely, from the uterus. Related to maternal hypertension, and the incidence increases with cocaine abuse. Partial detachment interferes with the functioning of the placenta, causing intrauterine growth restriction. Severe bleeding occurs with total detachment.	
Placenta previa	Placenta implants over or near the internal cervical opening. Implantation may be complete (covering the entire opening), partial, or marginal (to the edge of the cervical opening). Results in increased incidences of hemorrhage in the third trimester. Symptoms include painless bleeding after the 20th week of gestation.	Provide supportive care. Manage the patient's airway/ventilation/oxygen supplementation (100%). Transport rapidly if there is severe bleeding, high BP ≥160/110, seizures, or altered mental status.
Pregnancy-induced hypertension/ Preeclampsia/ Eclampsia	Hypertension >140/90 associated with increased protein in the urine and edema (peripheral or generalized) or an increase of ≥5 pounds of weight in one week after the 20th week of gestation. Severe preeclampsia is BP ≥160/110. Symptoms include headache, abdominal pain, and visual disturbances. May progress to eclampsia (seizures) and death.	

COMPLICATIONS OF DELIVERY

Complication	Characteristic	Prehospital
Cephalic (vertex) presentation	<u>Military</u>: Head straight, neck not flexed. <u>Brow</u>: Neck extended, brow presents first, can cause birth trauma so episiotomy or cesarean section (C-section) is usually required. <u>Face</u>: Severely extended neck with face presentation, may prolong labor, increase swelling of the fetus, and cause neck trauma.	Provide supportive care. Manage the patient's airway/ventilation/oxygen supplementation (100%). Transport rapidly.

Complication	Characteristic	Prehospital
Breech presentation	Frank breech (buttocks presentation with legs extended upward) is the most common, but single- or double-footling breech (incomplete breech) or buttocks presentation with legs flexed (complete breech) can also occur. Breech presentation is most common with placenta previa, hydramnios, fetal anomalies, and multiple gestations. Cord prolapse is more likely. Head trauma may occur because molding does not occur, and the head can become entrapped.	

PROLAPSE OF THE UMBILICAL CORD

A **prolapse of the umbilical cord** occurs when the umbilical cord precedes the fetus in the birth canal and becomes entrapped by the descending fetus. With an occult cord prolapse, the umbilical cord is beside or just ahead of the fetal head. With a nuchal cord prolapse, the cord tightly wraps about the fetal neck. About half of prolapses occur in the second stage of labor and relate to premature delivery, multiple gestations, or other complications. As contractions occur and the head descends, pressure to the umbilical cord occludes the blood flow, causing hypoxia and bradycardia. The decrease in blood flow through the umbilical vessels can cause impaired gas exchange, and if pressure on the cord is not relieved, the fetus can suffer severe neurological damage or death. Prehospital: Elevate the presenting part off the cord, slip the cord off of the fetus's neck if possible, elevate the mother's knees to the chest to relieve pressure on the cord, provide 100% oxygen, and transport rapidly.

INITIAL CARE OF THE NEWBORN

Dr. Virginia Apgar developed the **APGAR assessment** in 1952. APGAR stands for **a**ppearance, **p**ulse, **g**rimace, **a**ctivity, and **r**espiration. The APGAR is the first test given to a newborn. It is used as a quick evaluation of a newborn's physical condition to determine if any emergency medical care is needed, and it is administered 1 minute and 5 minutes after birth. The test is administered more than once because the baby's condition may change rapidly. It may be administered for a third time 10 minutes after birth, if needed. The baby is rated on the five subscales, and the scores are added together. A total score of ≥7 is a sign of good health.

APGAR ASSESSMENT

Sign	0	1	2
Appearance (skin color)	Cyanotic or pallor over entire body	Normal, except for the extremities	Entire body is normal.
Pulse (heart rate)	Absent	<100 bpm	>100 bpm.
Grimace (reflex irritability)	Unresponsive	Grimace	Infant sneezes, coughs, and recoils.
Activity (muscle tone)	Absent	Flexed limbs	Infant moves freely.
Respiration (breathing rate and effort)	Absent	Bradypnea, dyspnea	Good breathing and crying.

ROUTINE CARE OF THE NEWBORN

The infant should be given a **rapid assessment** within seconds of birth to determine if he or she is at term, if the amniotic fluid is clear, if there is muscle tone, and if there are respirations or crying. If any of these conditions are not met, then further resuscitation is needed. The basic steps to care include the following:

- Warming the infant after drying.
- Positioning the infant and clearing the airway if necessary.
- Stimulating and repositioning the infant.

The child should be evaluated throughout the initial procedures as follows:

- Respirations: The rate and character of the respirations should be noted as well as an observation of chest wall movement.
- Heart rate: Should be >100 bpm, assessed with a stethoscope or at the base of the umbilical cord.

Infants have poor temperature regulation ability, particularly preterm infants who lack brown fat, which is one of the body's tools to regulate body temperature, so **providing warmth** is critical as a component of resuscitation. An infant who is just seconds old and wet will need aggressive measures to keep him or her warm while any resuscitation efforts are being initiated. Infants lose heat through their heads, so one of the first steps should be to place a hat on the head or cover the head in some way. The infant should be vigorously dried with warmed blankets. Often, this stimulation—drying and warming—is all that is needed to establish a regular respiration pattern in the neonate. Preterm infants weighing <1500 grams should be placed in a plastic bag (made specifically for this purpose), if available, up to the height of the shoulders to prevent cold shock. A term infant with no apparent distress can be placed on the mother's chest and covered with a warm blanket.

To **establish an airway**, the infant is placed supine with the head slightly extended in the "sniffing" position. A small neck roll may be placed under the shoulders to maintain this position in a very small premature infant. Once the proper position is established, the mouth and nose are suctioned (suction the mouth first to prevent reflex inspiration of secretions when the nose is suctioned) with a bulb syringe or catheter if necessary. The infant's head can be turned momentarily to the side to allow secretions to pool in the cheek where they can be more easily suctioned and removed to establish the airway. **Stimulating** the newborn is often all that is needed to initiate spontaneous respirations. This tactile stimulation can be accomplished by gently rubbing the back or trunk of the infant. Another technique that is used to provide stimulation is flicking or rubbing the soles of the feet. Slapping neonates as stimulation is no longer practiced and should NOT be used.

Pediatric Considerations

Pediatric patients have the following general considerations:

- Proportionately greater body surface area to body mass ratio, so they are at greater risk of fluid and heat loss, burns, and absorption of toxins.
- Higher respiratory rates and heart rates than adults, resulting in higher oxygen demand.
- Immature blood/brain barrier, resulting in more neurological symptoms.
- Immature immune system, resulting in a higher risk of infection.
- Narrower and shorter airway and smaller jaw, so the tongue may easily obstruct the airway.
- Soft tracheal cartilage that increases the risk of airway collapse, large epiglottis.
- More pliable ribs, which provide less protection for abdominal organs, which are more forward.
- Liver and spleen that are proportionately larger and at risk of injury.
- Bones that are softer with open growth plates: An open growth plate injury can impair growth.
- Less protection for the brain and spinal cord (increasing the risk of injury) and less subarachnoid space.
- Cerebral blood-flow needs twice that of adults, increasing the risk of hypoxia.
- Limited glucose stores and risk of hypothermia (especially in the first month).
- Anterior fontanel that closes by 12 months and posterior fontanel that closes by 3–4 months.

Pediatric Assessment

Pediatric assessment should include the following:

- Pediatric assessment triangle:
    - Appearance (abnormal tone, decreased interactivity, decreased consolability, abnormal look/gaze, and abnormal speech or cry).

- o Work of breathing (abnormal sounds [wheezing, stridor], position, retractions [sternum], flaring [nostrils], and apnea/gasping).
- o Circulation (pallor, mottling, and cyanosis).
- Assess airway, breathing, and circulation (heart rate/pulse): Place in the shock position and provide a warming blanket for signs of shock.
- Ventilation/oxygenation: Administer oxygen and assist with ventilation if it is abnormal.
- Determine the patient's level of consciousness: Use the alert, voice, pain, unresponsive (AVPU) assessment. Note movement of the extremities and whether the pupils are normal, dilated, constricted, reactive, or fixed.
- Prevent hypothermia: Cover with a warming blanket, cover the head, and avoid unnecessary exposure of the skin.
- Obtain the medical history from the caregiver/parent: Include the type and duration of symptoms, fever, level of activity, recent foods/fluids, medications, medication allergies, past or chronic illnesses, and events leading to the current problem.
- Head-to-toe physical examination: Note any bruising, swelling, drainage, loose teeth, unusual odors, bleeding, rashes, deformities, and pain on movement.

PEDIATRIC SEIZURES

Febrile seizure is a generalized seizure associated with fever (usually >38.8°C [101.8°F]) from any type of infection (upper respiratory, urinary tract) but without intracranial infection or other cause, occurring between 6 months and 5 years of age. Seizures usually last <15 minutes and are without subsequent neurological deficit. Prehospital: Provide fever control (acetaminophen OR ibuprofen) and a tepid-water bath.

Other types of seizures may result from pathology, such as meningitis, cerebral edema, brain trauma, or brain tumors, but most seizures in children >3 are related to idiopathic epilepsy, which predisposes the child to recurrent seizures, usually of the same type. Seizures are characterized as focal (localized), focal with rapid generalization (spreading), and generalized (widespread). In most children, seizures become generalized with loss of consciousness. Seizure disorders with onset younger than 4 years of age usually cause more neurological damage than those with onset at older than 4 years of age. Prehospital: Place the patient on the floor or on a safe surface, loosen clothes, and protect him or her from injury during seizure. Afterwards, place the patient in the recovery position, monitor the airway/ventilation, and provide oxygen supplementation (the patient may need assisted ventilation if he or she is cyanotic) and suction if needed.

GROWTH AND DEVELOPMENT OF PEDIATRIC PATIENTS

Age	Characteristics
0–2 mos.	Sleeps up to 16 hours a day but should rouse easily. Cries for a reason; persistent crying may indicate illness. Limited head control. Gazes at faces.
2–6 mos.	Smiles voluntarily and makes eye contact, uses both hands, begins to hold head up, rolls over, and sleeps through the night.
6–12 mos.	Sits, crawls, has pincer grasp, mouths objects (increasing risk of poisoning and aspiration), babbles, and speaks first words by 12 months. Exhibits separation anxiety from parents.
12–18 mos.	Begins to walk; imitates others; knows body parts and 4–6 words; lacks molars for grinding food, increasing the risk of aspiration; and has increased mobility.
18–24 mos.	Begins to run and climb, knows 100 words (24 months), clings to parents, attaches to special objects, labels objects, and begins to understand cause and effect.
2–5 years	Walks, runs, throws, catches, is toilet trained, has magical thinking and irrational fears, learns acceptable behavior, has temper tantrums, and develops modesty.
6–12 years	Loses baby teeth; thinks logically; becomes self-conscious; understand the finality of death; attaches importance to school, popularity, and peers.
12–20 years	Puberty begins, reasons (imperfectly), is self-conscious, seeks independence and peer approval, and takes risks.

Apparent Life-Threatening Events (ALTES) and Sudden Infant Death Syndrome (SIDS)

Infants with an **apparent life-threatening event (ALTE)** are those who are lifeless and without respirations but are successfully resuscitated or begin breathing spontaneously. With **sudden infant death syndrome (SIDS),** which is almost always related to respiratory arrest, the child cannot be resuscitated. There are numerous proposed causes for ALTE and SIDS, so a careful history, including familial history of SIDS, and physical examination or postmortem examination can provide important information, such as indications of child abuse or metabolic/infectious disorders. Prehospital: Continue resuscitative efforts (airway/ventilation/oxygen supplementation, compressions as indicated) and stabilize the infant if possible. The child with ALTE should be hospitalized for observation, further studies, and apnea monitoring because these children are at an increased risk for SIDS. For SIDS patients, the paramedic should provide support and information to the family. The protocol for reporting SIDS varies by state, but it usually involves notifying the coroner's office.

Geriatric Considerations

Geriatric patients may have the following considerations:

- Decreased sensory input (hearing, vision, touch, pain); impaired depth perception and night vision; and decreased ability to differentiate colors.
- Hypertension, increasing the risk of heart attack and stroke.
- Decreased breathing capacity and decreased cough, increasing the risk of infection.
- Difficulty chewing and swallowing; digestive problems; and reflux when lying flat, increasing the risk of aspiration.
- Short-term memory deficit and slower reflexes.
- Decreased bone density, increasing the risk of breaks; loss of muscle tone.
- Increased risk of infection and less obvious symptoms of infection.
- Arthritis in the neck, interfering with airway assessment.
- Dentures that can obstruct the airway (leave them in place if possible during ventilation).
- Skin that is fragile and tears easily.
- Irregular pulse from underlying heart problems.
- Dementia (incidence increases with age), making history taking and treatment difficult.
- Atypical symptoms for illnesses, even if severely ill.
- Multiple comorbidities and multiple medications.
- Shock with BP greater than 100.

Delirium

Delirium is an acute sudden change in consciousness, characterized by reduced ability to focus or sustain attention, language and memory disturbance, disorientation, confusion, audiovisual hallucinations, sleep disturbance, and psychomotor activity disorder. Delirium differs from disorders with similar symptoms in that delirium is fluctuating. Delirium occurs in 10%–40% of hospitalized older adults and about 80% of patients who are terminally ill. Delirium may result from drugs such as anticholinergics and numerous conditions including infection, hypoxia, trauma, dementia, depression, vision and hearing loss, surgery, alcoholism, untreated pain, fluid/electrolyte imbalance, and malnutrition. Delirium increases the risks of morbidity and death, especially if untreated. Asking the patient to count backward from 20 to 1 and spell his or her first name backward can identify an attention deficit. Prehospital: Ensure the patient's safety, manage the patient's airway/ventilation/oxygen supplementation, and reorient the patient frequently.

Dementia

Type of dementia	Characteristics
Alzheimer's	Progressive dementia beginning with short-term memory loss and difficulty remembering names. It progresses to impaired judgment; disorientation; confusion; behavioral changes; difficulty understanding, reading, and using language; dysphagia; incoordination and inability to walk; and incontinence.
Creutzfeldt-Jakob disease	Rapidly progressive prion disease with impaired memory, behavioral changes, and incoordination, leading to death.
Huntington's disease	Progressive genetic disorder characterized by involuntary movements, muscle rigidity, abnormal eye movement, ataxia, lack of impulse and behavioral control, increasing confusion, difficulty communicating, and depression.
Pick's disease (frontotemporal dementia)	Form of progressive dementia resulting in destruction of neurons with change of personality and lack of judgment and empathy. Loss of language may include ability to understand and communicate.
Wernicke's encephalopathy	Inflammatory hemorrhagic encephalopathy due to thiamine deficiency, often associated with alcoholism. Symptoms include paralyzed eye muscles; double vision; ataxia; and a range of mental changes from forgetfulness to delirium tremens and Korsakoff's psychosis, which can lead to amnesia, disorientation, and hallucinations. Patients are able to produce language, although with some impairment, such as incorrect words or sounds, but they may have difficulty understanding.

Elder Abuse

Physical	Various types of assault related to hitting, kicking, pulling hair, shoving, and pushing. Patients may be forcibly confined, forced into seclusion, and/or force-fed to the point that they choke on food.
Psychological	Caregivers may threaten to hit the patient, brandish a weapon, and/or tell the person to commit suicide. Ongoing intimidation may make the patient terrified and anxious. Sometimes, caregivers threaten to injure pets or family members, increasing the patient's fear.
Sexual	Types of sexual abuse include the following: Physical: Fondling, kissing, and rape. Emotional: Exhibitionism. Verbal: Sexual harassment, using obscene language, and threatening.
Financial	Financial abuse includes the following: Outright stealing of property or persuading patients to give away possessions. Forcing patients to sign away property. Emptying bank and savings accounts and using stolen credit cards. Convincing the person to invest money in fraudulent schemes. Taking money for home renovations that are not done.

Child Abuse

Children rarely admit to **abuse** (physical, sexual, or emotional) and often attempt to protect the abusing parent. Therefore, suspicion of abuse depends on other indicators such as the following:

- **Behavioral:** The child may be overly compliant or fearful with obvious changes in demeanor when a parent/caregiver is present. Some children act out with aggression toward other children or animals. Children may become depressed or suicidal or present with sleeping or eating disorders. Behaviors may become increasingly self-destructive as the child ages, including inappropriate sexualized behavior.

- **Physical/Sexual:** The type, location, and extent of injuries can raise the suspicion of abuse. Head and facial injuries and bruising are common, as are bite or burn marks and spiral fractures. There may be handprints or grab marks and unusual bruising, such as across the buttocks. Any bruising, swelling, or tearing of the genital area and the identification of sexually transmitted diseases are also causes for concern.

Suspected abuse must be reported to the appropriate authorities, according to protocol, with careful documentation of findings and statements by the child or caregivers.

NEGLECT AND LACK OF SUPERVISED CARE

Children and older or impaired adults may suffer from profound **neglect or a lack of supervision** that places them at risk. Indicators include the following:

- Appearing dirty and unkempt, sometimes with infestations of lice, and wearing ill-fitting, torn clothing and shoes.
- Being tired and sleepy during the daytime.
- Having excessive medical or dental problems, such as extensive dental caries.
- Missing doctor appointments and not receiving proper immunizations.
- Being underweight for their current stage of development.
- Lacking assistive devices or misplaced hearing aids/eyeglasses.
- Left in soiled or urine-/feces-soiled clothing.
- Clothing is inadequate (such as lack of a coat/sweater during winter or dirty, torn, ill-fitting clothes).

Neglect can be difficult to assess, especially if the AEMT is serving a homeless or very disadvantaged population. Home visits may be needed to ascertain if there is adequate food, clothing, or supervision, and this is beyond the scope of care provided by the AEMT. Thus, suspicions should be reported to the appropriate authorities who can arrange a follow-up assessment of the home environment.

INJURIES CONSISTENT WITH DOMESTIC VIOLENCE/ABUSE

Characteristic injuries	Ruptured eardrum. Rectal/genital injury—burns, bites, trauma. Scrapes and bruises about the neck, face, head, trunk, arms. Cuts, bruises, and fractures of the face.
Patterns of injuries	"Bathing suit" pattern—injuries on parts of body that are usually covered with clothing because the perpetrator wants to hide the evidence of abuse. Head and neck injuries (50%).
Abusive injuries (rarely attributable to accidents)	Bites, bruises, rope and cigarette burns, and welts in the outline of weapons (belt marks). Bilateral injuries of the arms/legs.
Defensive injuries	Back-of-the-body injury from being attacked while crouched on the floor facedown. Located on the soles of the feet from kicking at a perpetrator. Located on the ulnar aspect of the hands or palm from blocking blows.

PATIENTS WITH SPECIAL CHALLENGES

Condition	Issues	Prehospital considerations
Homeless/ Indigent	Patients often are without medical care, increasing the risk of disease, and they may lack insurance. They may have mental health/substance abuse problems.	Know who will treat indigent patients and what resources are available in the community.

Condition	Issues	Prehospital considerations
Bariatric	Increased risk of chronic disease. Patients pose handling/moving problems and require special bariatric equipment and multiple personnel to assist. Patients often have trouble breathing and must have their head elevated.	Recognize the need for bariatric equipment and know how/where to obtain it. Notify the receiving facility. Use properly sized equipment, such as BP cuffs.
Technology-/Device-assisted	Wide range of issues including ventilators, apnea monitors, vascular devices, dialysis shunts, colostomies, ileostomies, and feeding tubes. Patients may have special needs regarding care and transport.	Ask about the patient's equipment and needs. Avoid disturbing/damaging the devices if possible.

EMS Operations

APPARATUS AND EQUIPMENT READINESS

The AEMT should ensure that the ambulance is ready for use and that the tires are properly inflated, the gas tank is full, warning devices are working, and engine fluid levels are appropriate. All necessary safety equipment, such as PPE (masks, gowns, gloves, and goggles or face guards) and safety devices (safety vests, road flares, and signs) as well as seat belts and harnesses, should be available and in proper working condition. All equipment in the cab, the compartments, and the rear of the ambulance should be in the proper place, labeled, and secured to prevent shifting during transportation. High-risk situations include going through intersections, inclement weather (especially with poor visibility), careless drivers, highway access, unpaved roads, and driver distractions (conversation, eating, drinking, mobile devices, music, GPS devices, and fatigue). During transportation, all personnel as well as patients should be properly secured with safety equipment.

SCENE-OF-INCIDENT SAFETY CONSIDERATIONS

The AEMT must do a 360° **assessment of the scene** of incident on arrival and determine safety considerations. The AEMT should make note of any gunshots heard, downed power lines, buildings in a state of collapse, leaking fuels/fluids, fire, smoke, broken glass, and other hazards. The AEMT may need to wait until the site is safe to proceed. The AEMT should assess the mechanism of injury (accidents) and the need for appropriate PPE (gloves, gown, mask, face guard) and must keep the patient informed of all actions and prevent harm or further injury. The ambulance should be parked off of the roadway if possible or parked at a 45° angle (front wheels out) to shield the work area, making sure not to block access for other emergency vehicles. Parking uphill is safer than downhill and upwind rather than downwind. If flares are used to warn other drivers, they should extend at least 300 feet from a collision. Yellow warning lights at the scene are the safest, but excessive lighting may blind other drivers at night.

TRANSFERRING A PATIENT FROM THE SCENE TO AN AMBULANCE

Different types of **stretchers** and **transfer equipment** may be used for prehospital transfer, including the following:

- Wheeled: Stretcher that can be lowered and raised with a wheeled base allowing it to slide into the ambulance.
- Scoop: Two- to four-piece stretcher that can be connected and placed under a patient.
- Transfer sheet: A heavy plastic sheet can be used with patients up to 800 lb to facilitate transfer.
- Flexible stretcher: Lightweight flexible (plastic, rubberized canvas) stretcher with webbing handles on both sides. Can be used to transfer patients around corners and up and down stairs where a wheeled stretcher cannot be used.
- Stair chair: Safety chair that can be used to transfer patients in tight spaces and up and down stairs.
- Lightweight stretcher: Folding stretcher made of lightweight materials.
- Basket stretcher (Stokes basket): Used primarily for rescues in the wilderness or from cliffs.

Patient positioning should be according to the possible or probable injury, with safety restraints always securing the patient to the gurney and the gurney to the vehicle.

- Left-side-lying: Pregnant patients should be placed in this position to increase circulation to the placenta, and unconscious patients should be placed in this position to prevent aspiration and choking if there is no indication of a spinal injury.
- Supine (flat on the back): Patient has a suspected pelvic fracture or neck injury (also requires a cervical collar).
- Supine (feet elevated above the heart): This is the position for patients in shock to increase circulation to the heart and brain as the BP falls.

- <u>Trendelenburg</u> (the entire stretcher is tilted so that the head is below the feet): Position for patients with a suspected spinal cord injury.
- <u>Semi-Fowler's</u> (30- to 45-degree position): For patients with chest pain, stroke, and/or shortness of breath and no indication of a spinal cord injury.
- <u>Fowler's</u> (upright, 90-degree position): For patients with severe shortness of breath.

ENVIRONMENTAL RISK FACTORS

When assessing a patient, it's important to consider that **environmental factors** may place the patient at an increased risk for harm or may be a factor in disease. There are a number of different types of environmental factors to consider.

Factors	Examples	Effects
Toxic chemicals	Lead, arsenic, muriatic acid, sulfuric acid, ammonia, lime	May result in poisoning (lead, arsenic) or burns (acids, ammonia, lime) through direct exposure or inhalation
Physical objects	Guns, cars, knives, equipment	Accidents, gunshot wounds, stabbings, various injuries (blunt and penetrating)
Biological organisms	Bacteria, fungi, viruses	Infections
Temperature variations	Heat, cold	Burns, dehydration, heat stroke, hyperthermia, hypothermia, frostbite
Ambient noise	Sirens, loud music, traffic noise, work-related noise	Hearing loss/deafness, increased anxiety
Psychosocial	Increased stress	Anxiety, hypertension, suicidal ideation

RESCUES IN CONFINED SPACES

A **confined space** is one in which access is limited and the space is surrounded by walls or structures that are not suitable for habitation. A confined space may occur in a building (such as with a collapse), a silo, a motor vehicle (such as a large vehicle involved in a crash), a cistern or septic tank, or a well. A confined space may pose a risk to the patient and the AEMT because of difficulty moving about and accessing the patient as well as decreased ventilation that may result in the buildup of toxic gases and/or a lack of oxygen. Before entering a confined space, the AEMT should test the atmosphere and use the correct breathing equipment. This is especially important if the patient is nonresponsive, which is often an indication of poor air quality. The AEMT should also carefully assess his or her ability to access the patient and the best means of doing so.

DRIVING SAFETY

The **ambulance driver** should stop briefly or slow significantly at intersections because other drivers may not hear or may ignore sirens. The driver should keep the brake covered with the left foot for fast braking and avoid excessive speeds because of the increased risk of accidents, especially on curves. The speed should be adjusted for road and weather conditions and should not be influenced by use of the siren (siren syndrome). Snow and ice should be cleared from the ambulance before driving it. At least one vehicle length should separate the ambulance from other vehicles for every 10 mph of speed. A spotter should always be used when backing up the ambulance because of poor visibility. All personnel in the ambulance should be seated and secured with seat belts or safety harnesses before the ambulance moves. Studies have shown that CPR is most effective if done from a sitting position in an ambulance rather than standing, despite common practice. Patients and gurneys should also be secured.

LIGHTS AND SIRENS

Lights and sirens should be used together, and they are indicated when going to a scene and when transporting a patient in a serious emergent situation. There are four types of warning lights used on emergency vehicles such as ambulances: rotating lights (resulting in a flashing sensation), fixed flashes (usually red or blue), strobe lights, and LED lights. Red (the most common) and blue lights are generally used to indicate emergency vehicles and can be used to obtain the right-of-way or to block the right-of-way. These colors may be interchangeable, although in some states the color blue is restricted to law enforcement vehicles. Amber lights are warning lights and can be used by all vehicles, but they do not require others to stop. Some emergency vehicle lights change to amber when the vehicle is parked. White warning lights cannot be used on the rear of an emergency vehicle. Green lights are sometimes used to indicate a mobile incident command post, but in some states, green lights may also indicate private security vehicles or volunteer firefighters.

INCIDENT MANAGEMENT

FEMA IS-700.A outlines the **National Incident Management System (NIMS)**, which, under the direction of the Federal Emergency Management Agency (FEMA), an agency of the US Department of Homeland Security, provides the foundation for collaboration among different governmental and nongovernmental agencies, jurisdictions, and specialties/disciplines in handling large-scale incidents that threaten life, property, and/or the environment. Components of FEMA IS-700.A include the following:

- Preparedness: Focuses on planning, procedures and protocols, training and exercises, personnel qualifications/certification, and equipment certification, and it includes the National Response Framework, which ensures that local jurisdictions retain control but use a unified approach and establishes protocols.
- Communications and information management: Systems must be interoperable, reliable, portable, scalable, resilient, and redundant.
- Resource management: Includes personnel, equipment, supplies, and facilities, which must be inventoried and categorized using a standardized approach.
- Command and management: Includes the Incident Command System (this standardized approach outlines the responsibilities of the incident commander, area command, command staff, and general staff), multiagency coordination systems, and public information.
- Management and maintenance: The National Integration Center (NIC) is responsible for NIMS.
- Flexibility: Components are scalable and adaptable to all types of incidents.
- Standardization: The NIC develops standards in cooperation with standards development organizations.

ICS-100.B, the **Incident Command System** course, meets NIMS requirements for operational personnel and outlines a standardized approach to incident management. ICS is used for any type of major event, planned or otherwise, and large- or small-scale incidents, including natural (disasters), technological (hazmat release), and human-caused (civil disturbance) hazards. ICS outlines the chain of command (the incident commander in control and orders going through supervisors). Every incident requires an incident action plan, resource management, and processes for reimbursement. The incident commander establishes an incident command post and staging areas (gathering places) as well a base (coordination area for logistic and administrative functions), camps (for sleeping, eating, and sanitary services), helibases, and helispots. Primary features of ICS include common terminology, establishment/transfer of command, chain of command/unity of command, management of objects, incident action planning, modular organization, manageable span of control, comprehensive resource management, incident facilities and locations, integrated communications, information and intelligence management, accountability, and dispatch/deployment.

CHAIN OF COMMAND/UNITY OF COMMAND/UNIFIED COMMAND

Each organization must establish the **chain of command** for its incident command system. Although these may vary somewhat, an incident commander is ultimately in charge with individuals being assigned as incident managers in different areas, such as triage, treatment, transport, security, and liaison. **Unity of command** means that each incident commander should have control over personnel assigned to his or her area, and each individual within the chain of command should have a clear understanding of whom to report to at the scene so that communication is efficient and timely. **Unified command** means that when multiple agencies are involved from multiple jurisdictions, the chain of command that has been established is recognized and respected even though each agency retains its own authority and accountability and is responsible for carrying out its own duties. A unified command system prevents duplication of effort as well as neglect of important functions.

INCIDENT ACTION PLAN

The purpose of the **incident action plan** is to outline control objectives, resources, and strategies for dealing with an incident. Incident action plans should be updated frequently. Incident action plans may be designed for various types of incidents (terrorist attack, disease outbreak, hurricane) and modified as needed and should include the following:

- Goals and objectives, including expected outcomes.
- Strategies and tactics for responding and accomplishing the goals and objectives.
- An outline of the chain of command for the incident command system, including the span of control (the number of people reporting to an individual).
- Tasks assigned to each level in the chain of command.
- Safety/Health plan for responders to prevent injury/illness and to treat as needed.
- Communications plan outlining how information will be exchanged, including alternative methods of command if, for example, cell phone towers are out of commission.
- Logistics plan regarding the acquisition and use of resources, such as supplies, personnel, and equipment.
- Maps and demographic information.

INCIDENT COMMANDER

When a multiple-casualty or mass-casualty event occurs, the first lead emergency medical responder on the scene generally assumes the role of **incident commander** and carries out a rapid assessment of the scene and begins to call for additional resources as indicated while another medical responder begins triage. The incident commander should begin to establish a command center in an area that is safe and out of the way of emergency vehicles while awaiting assistance. This first incident commander will relinquish the role when the staffed and/or assigned incident commander arrives to take command and should then report to the person who is assuming the role of staging officer. The incident commander's duties include establishing command, assessing needs, developing a plan, coordinating all activities, delegating responsibilities, ensuring the safety of all personnel and patients, liaising with other agencies, and communicating information.

PRIMARY TRIAGE AND RESOURCE MANAGEMENT

Primary triage is a rapid method (30–60 seconds) of prioritizing patients based on the severity of their condition, and it is carried out at the scene of multiple-casualty incidents. All patients are triaged and tagged according to the following international color-coding priority (P) guidelines on the foot or wrist (not on the clothing):

- P1—Red: Immediate care is needed for urgent systemic life-threatening conditions, such as airway/breathing problems, severe bleeding, severe burns (especially with breathing problems), decreased mental status, shock, and severe medical problems, or a Glasgow Coma Scale score of ≤13.
- P2—Yellow: Delayed care and able to wait 45–60 minutes for treatment. Conditions include burns (without breathing problems), multiple bone/joint injuries, back and/or spinal cord injuries (unless the patient is in respiratory distress).
- P3—Green: Hold, able to wait hours for treatment of minor injuries.
- P4—Black: Deceased.

Resource management involves identifying a triage officer, who remains at the scene during the event and identifying the need for additional personnel and equipment and providing those to the patients with the highest priority.

SECONDARY TRIAGE/RETRIAGE

During a mass-casualty incident, triage is done quickly, and patients may be scattered over a wide area with many patients being red-tagged for emergency care. Patients coded black are left in place, but those with other-color tags should be moved and segregated in separate sections of a holding area to await treatment and/or transport. The patients should be **retriaged** as they are moved into the holding area to determine if the tagging color is still appropriate. Additionally, **secondary triage** may be carried out in the separate sections, especially if some must be airlifted, to determine which patients have the best chance of survival and should receive priority for transfer and treatment. Secondary triage may also help to determine which trauma center (based on location or level of care) or hospital is most appropriate for the patient considering the patient's condition, transport time, and the surge capacity of the healthcare institutions.

CENTERS FOR DISEASE CONTROL AND PREVENTION GUIDELINES FOR FIELD TRIAGE OF INJURED PATIENTS

The **CDC's guidelines for field triage** of injured patients is a four-step algorithm that is used to identify the most seriously ill patients and transport them to an appropriate treatment center.

Step	Assess	Findings requiring priority treatment	Plan
1	Vital signs/Level of consciousness	Glasgow Coma Scale score of ≤13, systolic BP <90 mm Hg, respiratory rate <10 or >29 per minute (<20 in an infant <1 year), or need of ventilatory support.	Highest level trauma center
2	Anatomy of injury	Penetrating injuries, flail chest, two or more long-bone fractures, crushed/mangled/pulseless extremity, amputations, pelvic fractures, open/depressed skull fracture, or paralysis.	Highest level trauma center
3	Mechanism of injury/High-energy impact	Falls—adults >20 feet and children >10 feet or 2–3 times their height. High-risk auto crash with intrusions, partial or complete ejection, or there is a death in the same passenger compartment. Auto vs. pedestrian/bicycle with victim thrown, run over, or sustaining a significant impact. Motorcycle crash >20 mph.	Trauma center
4	Special patient/system considerations	Older adults, children, pregnancy >30 weeks, burns, patients on anticoagulants or with bleeding disorders (based on the AEMT's best judgment).	Trauma center/Hospital

START METHOD OF TRIAGE

With the **START method of triage**, the paramedic starts triage with the first victim encountered, tags the patient, and then moves to the next patient, assessing in order: (1) respirations, (2) perfusion, and (3) mental status (RPM) and using the standard red-yellow-green-black color-coding system. Walking wounded are tagged as green.

Respirations	Present.	Red tag if >30. Continue to perfusion assessment if <30.
	Not present—position the airway.	Red tag if respirations recur or black tag (death) if none.
Perfusion	Radial pulse absent or capillary refill of greater than 2 seconds.	Control bleeding and red tag.
	Radial pulse present and capillary refill time of less than 2 seconds.	Continue to mental status assessment.
	Cannot follow simple directions.	Red tag.

Mental status	Can follow simple directions.	Yellow tag.

JumpSTART Method of Triage for Pediatric Patients

JumpSTART is a pediatric triage method developed only for use in multiple-casualty incidents.

Able to walk	No	Continue to breathing assessment.
	Yes	Green tag. Carry out secondary triage.
Breathing	No	Step 1: Position upper airway and red tag if breathing. Step 2: Give five rescue breaths and red tag if breathing. Black tag if breathing does not recur.
	Yes	Respiratory rate <15 or >45, red tag. Respiratory rate 15 to 45, continue to pulse assessment.
Palpable pulse	No	Red tag.
	Yes	Continue to AVPU assessment.
Alert, voice, pain, unresponsive (AVPU) assessment	Inappropriate pain, posturing, or unresponsive	Red tag.
	A, V, or P is appropriate	Yellow tag.

Critical Incident Stress Management (CISM)

Critical incident stress management (CISM) is a procedure to help people cope with stressful events, such as disasters, in order to reduce the incidence of post-traumatic stress syndrome (PTSS).

- Defusing sessions usually occur very early, sometimes during or immediately after a stressful event, and they are used to educate personnel who are actively involved about what to expect over the next few days and to provide guidance in handling their feelings and stress levels.
- Debriefing sessions usually follow in one to three days and may be repeated periodically as needed. These sessions may include people who were directly involved as well as those who were indirectly involved. People are encouraged to express their emotions about the event. Critiquing the event or attempting to place blame is not productive as part of the CISM process.
- Follow-up is done at the end of the process, usually after about week, but this time frame can vary.

Air Medical Transport

Air medical transport is indicated when the patient is in need of a high level of care that may be available on an aircraft but not an ambulance, when the patient's condition and need for treatment are time critical, when the patient is located in a remote area where access by ambulance is difficult or would be delayed (helicopter), or when local medical services have exceeded their capacity. Helipads are often available at large hospitals, so the patient can be treated immediately after arrival. Some disadvantages include inclement weather (which may interfere with flight plans) as well as altitude and airspeed limitations. Depending on the aircraft, the cabin size may be inadequate for the patient, personnel, and equipment. Difficult terrain, such as forested or hilly areas may not provide an adequate landing site. Cost is the biggest difference between ground and air transport with air transport often costing tens of thousands of dollars with only part, or in some cases none, of the costs being covered by insurance.

Helicopters have the advantage over fixed-wing aircraft of being able to load a patient at or near the scene rather than having to transport the patient by ambulance to an airport. A paved surface is not necessary for a helicopter landing site, but level grassy or paved sites are preferred, ideally with 100 × 100 feet of clear space, but a minimum area of 60 × 60 feet may be used. Additionally, the area should be free of debris that may be disrupted by the rotor blades and should be clear of structures that may interfere with the aircraft, such as power poles, tall trees, power lines, cables, and antennas. A rotor aircraft does not require that people approach in a crouching position, but people should avoid holding anything over their heads and should generally approach from the front of the aircraft and avoid the rear of the aircraft and the rear rotors.

The pilot in command (PIC) of rotorcraft and fixed-wing aircraft is responsible for the **safety** of the aircraft, crew, emergency medical personnel, and the patient. As with all takeoffs and landings, medical staff and crew must be seated and secured by seat belts. Helmets should be in place and secure. Patients who are violent, confused, or combative should be physically restrained for transport and may also require chemical restraints to ensure their own personal safety as well as the safety of the medical and flight crew. Patients should be offloaded ONLY when a crew member signals the receiving medical personnel to approach the aircraft. With high-altitude fixed-wing air transports, cabins are pressurized but only to the equivalent of 6000–8000 feet, not to sea level. Rotorcraft are usually used to transfer a patient from the scene of an incident to a primary care facility or from the primary care facility to another type of facility, whereas a fixed-wing aircraft is usually used from one facility to another over longer distances.

COMMUNICATION ISSUES ASSOCIATED WITH AIR MEDICAL SERVICES

A **communication specialist** should coordinate all air medical services, including communications within an agency and between agencies regarding all aspects of transport. The communication specialist should have radio communication skills and knowledge of medical terminology, including knowledge of how to obtain information about a patient, navigation, map usage, customer service, weather, aircraft emergencies, as well as FAA and Federal Communications Commission (FCC) regulations that relate to air medical transport. The communication specialist should be familiar with radio frequencies used by EMS. The dispatcher determines whether an aircraft should take off. The communication center may be located in a medical facility, airport, or other space, but it should be free of distractions and have emergency backup electrical power. All air medical transport team members should have knowledge of the radio communication system. Some systems include radio or radio-phone communication, and some systems require the team members to carry pagers, such as two-way satellite pagers. All incoming and outgoing communication should be recorded.

STATE AND FEDERAL REGULATIONS REGARDING AIR MEDICAL SERVICES

State **statutes** require that aircraft used for air ambulance service must be licensed to provide that service, and the service must ensure that all required medical equipment is available. Although statutes may vary slightly from one state to another, most require that the service be able to provide basic and advanced life support and should provide patients with a description of services and costs. Additionally, the aircraft and crew must comply with Federal Aviation Administration (FAA) regulations and carry insurance to cover injuries that may occur in transport. The FAA carries out periodic inspections of aircraft and issues resource documents regarding safety and operations. Federal regulations establish weather guidelines for safe flying. The US Department of Transportation provides guidelines regarding standards of care. The Commission on Accreditation of Medical Transport Systems establishes voluntary accreditation standards, but air medical services associated with hospitals must meet hospital accreditation standards, typically those of the Joint Commission.

SAFE EXTRICATION FROM A MOTOR VEHICLE (CAR, TRUCK)

Scene management at the site of an accident that requires vehicle extrication incudes initial evaluation of any hazards at the site (360° evaluation), such as oncoming traffic, fallen wires, spilled fuel, and fire/explosion risk or presence. The scene must be secured (45° parking, police security, flares, and cones) and the AEMT should don protective equipment as necessary and access the patient to provide life-saving care. The patient must be disentangled from the motor vehicle as much as can be done safely. The patient is prepared for extrication (such as by applying pressure to bleeding sites and placing a cervical collar), removed from the vehicle, and then prepared for ground or air transport and provided emergent treatment. For extrications in difficult terrain, assess the following:

- <u>Terrain</u>: Forests, desert, cliff, water, snow.
- <u>Obstacles</u>: Trees, rocks, light, unavailability of landing sites.
- <u>Methods to be used</u>: Helicopter extrication, overland carry, type of extrication.
- <u>Alternative solutions</u>: Abort; contact search and rescue.
- <u>Safety issues</u>: Review all safety concerns.

For **vehicle extrication,** the vehicle must be stabilized before the EMS personnel attempt to enter the vehicle or administer aid to the patient, especially if the vehicle may slide or is on its side and the personnel must access the vehicle from the top because the vehicle may shift and further endanger the patient as well as EMS personnel. EMS personnel can access the vehicle through a window (breaking it if necessary) or a door if one is operable (the patient may be able to assist in opening a window or door). EMS personnel should carry an airway (in case the patient requires ventilation), dressings (to apply pressure if the patient is bleeding), and a rigid cervical collar (to protect against spinal injury or further spinal damage) and should do rapid triage on access to the patient. Oxygen is usually not administered until after the patient is extracted because of the danger of fire, especially if the patient is saturated with fuel, and CPR is not done until the patient is in the supine position on a solid surface. If patients are apneic and pulseless, they must be removed as quickly as possible even with only manual protection of the spine being provided.

For **vehicle extrication**, once EMS personnel have gained access to the motor vehicle, they should unlock its doors if possible to allow others to more easily gain access. The EMS personnel should ensure that the engine is turned off, the parking brake is set, and the transmission is set to park. If possible, an emergency response person should disconnect the battery to decrease the risk of fire and explosion. If the patient can be removed, a short backboard should be applied before moving the patient. If the patient is wedged between the seat and the steering wheel, the seat may be slid back manually while rescuers support the patient. If the seat has become dislodged from the track, then the patient should be completely immobilized because this type of mechanical damage can result in severe physical injury. If the patient's legs are trapped, lifting the steering wheel away may also lift the dashboard and help to release the patient.

If a patient must be **cut from a vehicle** (such as when the vehicle is on its side and access must be through a U-shaped flap in the roof), he or she should be warned of the noise and should be covered with a safety blanket (heavy aluminized). In some accidents, **air bags** may not deploy, but movement of the patient or vehicle may cause them to deploy, resulting in danger to the patient and EMS personnel. If the air bags have not deployed, then the battery cables should be disconnected or cut (negative side first) to prevent deployment and personnel should avoid being in front of the path of deployment. EMS personnel should check for side air bags as well as front. The air bags should be deactivated before the steering column is moved (keeping in mind that deactivation can take up to 30 minutes), and care should be taken to avoid cutting or drilling into an air bag.

Since the 1990s, vehicles have been equipped with **seat belt pretensioners** on three-point (shoulder harness) systems in the front and often also in the back. The purpose of seat belt pretensioners is to tighten any slack in the belts in an accident, pulling the person back into the seat and in the proper position for deployment of the air bag. Evidence of pretensioners is not always visible, although an accordion sleeve near the buckle end may be an indication. This sleeve compresses if the pretensioner fires. Although an undeployed pretensioner poses less threat to EMS personnel than an undeployed air bag, it can increase the risk of injury to the patient or EMS personnel, so the seat belt should be disconnected or cut immediately on access to the patient. If the patient was not wearing the seat belt on impact and the pretensioner fired, the seat belt will be tightly vertical along pillar B. If the seat belt pretensioner fired while being worn, it will be extended and will not be retractable.

Although large and heavy pieces of equipment, such as hydraulic rescue tools (including the Jaws of Life, cutters, spreaders, truck jacks, and rams), pneumatic tools, and come-along tools, are often used in vehicle extrication, a tool kit with **simple hand tools** should also be readily available. They may also be needed to access and safely remove a patient from a vehicle. Tools that may be needed for disassembly include adjustable wrenches, screwdrivers (flat and Phillips), flashlight, penlight, medical scissors, headlamp, pliers, bolt cutters, hammers, axes, crowbars, rescue knives (specially designed to cut through seat belts and clothing), and tin snips. Combination rescue tools are available that can be used for a variety of purposes, such as shutting off gas valves, prying open windows, and cutting through battery cables. Tool belt pouches are available to hold small tools that may be needed during an extrication.

Cribbing and chocking are used to raise a vehicle and prevent it from rolling, such as when a patient is caught beneath a vehicle. Cribbing consists of 2×4 blocks and wedges and 4×4 blocks and wedges that are used to create crib boxes to hold an air bag. Cribs are usually made of Douglas fir or southern yellow pine, which can hold 500 psi and crushes slowly. The cribbing is stacked with a 4-inch overhang (to allow for compression), and it should not exceed 48 inches in height. The crib box is put in place with the air bag on top. Chocks are large stepped wedges that are placed in front of or behind wheels to keep them from rolling when the air bag is inflated. As the air bag is slowly inflated, capture cribbing stacks are placed on both sides behind it to hold the vehicle when the air bag is deflated. Once the vehicle is elevated and secured, the air bag is deflated and the crib box is removed to allow room for extrication of the patient.

Some vehicles are powered by **alternative fuels**, such as compressed natural gas (CNG) or liquefied natural gas (LNG), so EMS personnel should look for CNG/LNG logos, often on the right rear or near the refueling port or the right rear of the cab (semitruck). A "natural gas vehicle" warning may be located near the bottom of the rear doors. CNG tanks may be located behind the cabs in semitractors, and some may have additional saddle tanks. The power should be turned off, and the 12-volt battery positive and negative cables should be cut. The emergency shut-off valve should be located and turned off, although each tank can also be turned off manually. Electric vehicles pose the risk of stranded energy. Batteries should always be considered energized with a potential for high-voltage injury. Damaged lithium ion batteries that are leaking or sparking are at risk for thermal runaway (fire). The car battery should be shut down immediately. If the battery is damaged, the vehicle must be relocated at least 50 feet from any combustible material.

BUS EXTRICATION

Before accessing patients involved in a **bus crash,** the bus must be stabilized, especially if it is on its side or if it is upside down. If the engine is still running, a stop button is often located on the left side of the front panel. Access to the bus may be through the front door if possible. Access may also be through the front windshield (which can be removed through removal of the rubber locking strip that surrounds the window), side windows, the emergency exit door or window, the bathroom window, or an opening cut into the top of the vehicle. Removal of injured patients (usually on stretchers) from inside the vehicle often requires rapid triage and the assistance of multiple EMS personnel. If the vehicle remains upright but patients are completely or partially beneath the vehicle, they should be removed quickly because they may be crushed if the air suspension system deflates.

AIRCRAFT EXTRICATION

Communication is essential if EMS personnel are responding to an **aircraft crash site** because they need to know when the crash occurred, the type and size of the aircraft, the number of passengers and crew, reports of fire or explosion, and whether the aircraft is private, commercial, or military, as well as the status (fire, collapse) of any structure(s) that the aircraft may have impacted. For a small plane with the cabin still reasonably intact, extrication may be similar to a motor vehicle, but severe crashes in which the cabin is destroyed and large airplane crashes pose significantly different problems because passengers may have been thrown about inside or outside of the aircraft and seats and belongings and body parts may block access. Victims may lie in the roadway, so emergency vehicles must proceed with caution. Fire and explosions may be a severe risk, and rescuers may need to wait for fire suppression. Triage may begin outside of the aircraft while the aircraft (or the remains of the aircraft) is secured.

EXTRICATION CONSIDERATIONS

Part of the stabilization of the scene is ensuring that it is secure. An outer perimeter is established to block public and media access, and an inner perimeter is established immediately about the scene of the rescue and the working crew. Three **control zones** are established as follows:

- Hot (coded red): This encompasses the inner perimeter and the crew as well as any area that is dangerous, such as an area contaminated by hazardous material or one in danger of a release of toxins.
- Warm (coded orange): Area for trained personnel in support of those in the hot zone. Decontamination of patients, crew, and equipment is carried out in this zone.
- Cold (coded yellow): This is the staging area and the command post (if necessary for the emergent situation). No members of the public or media should be allowed in the cold zone.

Zones are usually established by placement of police cars and fire-line tape.

The **path of least resistance** is an important concept to understand for rescues, especially if they involve fire and any products of combustion (smoke, heat, gas). Fire's path of least resistance is usually vertical and upward, although fire also spreads horizontally, especially if a vertical path is not available. It's for this reason that if there is a fire on the top floor of a building, the roof is breached to prevent horizontal spread. External factors, such as gusts of wind, can affect the path of least resistance. Water, on the other hand, also flows vertically, but downward and then horizontally if the downward flow is blocked. If the AEMT is rescuing patients from a building, they will often be found near the path of least resistance, such as a near a door or window. Patients should also be transported according to the path of least resistance, that is, the route that is the easiest and safest.

MULTISTEP RESCUE PROCESS

The **multistep rescue process** includes the following 10 steps:

1. Preparation: Training, readying equipment, and preparing for different types of rescues.
2. Response: Using protocols for dispatch; contacting others, such as utility companies, which may have the necessary knowledge or equipment.
3. Situation size-up: 360° site survey to identify hazards and determine the need for additional personnel or equipment. Determine if the situation is rescuer/equipment intensive.
4. Stabilization: Establishing perimeters and control zones, monitoring hazardous atmosphere, carrying out lockout/tagout of industrial equipment.
5. Access: Gaining access to the patient and providing emergent care.
6. Disentanglement: Freeing the patient.
7. Removal: Continuing critical and life support while assisting the patient to move or carrying the immobilized patient. Rapid extraction if his or her condition is life threatening.
8. Transport: Transporting by various means with decontamination done as needed.
9. Scene security: Police or others providing protection of the scene, crew, and patients.
10. Postevent analysis: Reviewing the procedures performed and the problems encountered.

OCCUPATIONAL SAFETY AND HEALTH ADMINISTRATION (OSHA)

The **Occupational Safety and Health Administration** (OSHA) is part of the US Department of Labor, and it is charged with ensuring safe, healthful working conditions and setting and enforcing workplace standards. OSHA covers most employers in the private sector, but state and federal safety regulations also generally conform to OSHA standards. Employers must provide safety training, inform workers of chemical hazards, and provide required PPE. OSHA must be notified of a workplace-related death within 8 hours and a workplace-related injury that results in hospitalization, the loss of an eye, or amputation within 24 hours. Workers may file a complaint about workplace conditions with OSHA and request an inspection. OSHA's Whistleblower Protection Program prohibits retaliation by the employer. OSHA provides Hazardous Waste Operations and Emergency Response Standard (HAZWOPER) training courses (8-hour, 24-hour, 40-hour, and refresher) for first responders. OSHA has established regulations and guidelines that are industry specific. For example, OSHA has regulations regarding EMS. OSHA requires that hazardous material be color coded, with red indicating danger; yellow, caution; orange, warning; and fluorescent orange/orange-red, biological hazard.

> **Review Video: Intro to OSHA**
> Visit mometrix.com/academy and enter code: 913559

HAZARDOUS MATERIALS AND EXPOSURE

Hazardous materials are any that may cause harm to humans or animals by themselves or through interaction with something else. Hazardous materials may be any of the following:

- Chemical: Include blister agents, blood agents, choking agents, nerve agents, asphyxiants, and irritants. These can enter the body through inhalation, absorption, ingestion, and injection.
- Radiological: Nuclear material and radioactive substances (alpha/beta particles).
- Physical/Biological: Infectious wastes, blood and other body fluids, and biotoxins.

Almost any material or substance can be classified as hazardous depending on various factors such as its location, amount, and interactions. Exposure occurs when a person/animal comes in contact with the hazardous material, and contamination is the residue resulting from exposure. Absorption is the method by which hazardous material enters the bloodstream. Exposure and contamination may result in an immediate response (blistering, itching, and pain) or a delayed response (nausea, vomiting, cancer, and lung disease).

The Environmental Protection Agency (EPA) classifies **hazardous wastes** according to the following characteristics:

- Ignitable: Liquids and nonliquids that can ignite and cause fires with flash points of <60°C/140°F.
- Corrosive: Based on pH (<2 or >12.5) or its ability to corrode steel.
- Reactive: Wastes that are unstable, may react with water, or that may result in toxic gases. They may also explode.
- Toxic: Heavy metal compounds that are harmful if ingested or absorbed.

Wastes may also be classified as listed wastes. These include wastes from manufacturing and industrial processes. Hazardous wastes are often produced in manufacturing, nuclear power plants (nuclear wastes), and healthcare facilities (needles and materials contaminated with body fluids). Nuclear wastes are classified as mixed waste because they contain a radioactive component as well as a hazardous component. Hazardous wastes can result in disease (such as from needle punctures), injury (from fire and explosions), and death (from toxic exposure and disease).

The purpose of **hazardous waste site characterization** is to identify hazards and select the appropriate PPE. The team leader is responsible for the assessment, but he or she may request assistance from outside experts, such as chemists. The three steps to hazardous waste site characterization include the following:

1. Off-site characterization: Gather information/data before personnel enter the site, including the location, a description of the activities, the duration of the event, terrain information (photographs, maps), habitation/population data, accessibility, paths of least resistance, and properties of any hazardous materials/substances. Conduct the needed interviews and review of records. Perimeter reconnaissance is done with observations, air sampling, and development of a preliminary site map.
2. On-site survey: Verify the information gathered from perimeter reconnaissance, survey the area and situation, note potential exposure to hazardous materials (dust, liquid, dead animals, gas) and safety hazards (obstacles, terrain, poisonous plants), and develop a site safety plan. The entry team should have at least four members: two to enter and two for outside support who can enter the site in an emergency.
3. Ongoing monitoring: Monitoring should be continuous.

CHEMICAL HAZARDOUS WASTE MATERIALS

Types of **chemical hazardous waste materials** include the following:

- Blister agents: Include sulfur mustard (mustard gas) and nitrogen mustard, which are both highly toxic. Exposure by inhalation, contact, or ingestion results in skin (erythema and blistering) and eye irritation and injury to the respiratory system as well as bone marrow suppression and gastrointestinal and neurological damage. The patient should be decontaminated within 1 to 2 minutes by flushing the eyes with water for up to 20 minutes and removing clothing and showering with soap (if available) and water for 20 minutes. Rescuers should use a self-contained breathing apparatus (SCBA), PPE (including eye protection), and chemical-protective gloves.
- Asphyxiants: Gas exposure (such as by butane, helium, and propane) lowers oxygen levels and results in suffocation. Patients require oxygen administration and may need CPR. This is especially a risk in confined spaces. Rescuers should use an SCBA.
- Blood agents: These include cyanide chloride, hydrogen cyanide, and arsine. Exposure by inhalation or ingestion. They prevent oxygen transfer from blood to cells. The patient may need oxygen and antidote. Rescuers should use an SCBA.
- Carcinogens: Agents such as asbestos, nickel compounds, and ionizing radiation that result in genetic mutation and cancer. There are various types of exposure. Patients must be removed from exposure. The rescuer must wear adequate PPE, and in some cases, he or she should use a mask or SCBA.
- Choking agents: Often, a chemical weapon is used (ammonia, chlorine) that is designed to inhibit breathing and incapacitate the person. Exposure is by inhalation, contact, or ingestion (rare). They may be corrosive to the skin and result in fluid in the lungs, leading to suffocation. Patients require supportive treatment and oxygen. Rescuers should use PPE and SCBA for most agents.
- Convulsants/Nerve agents: These include hydrazine and strychnine. Exposure may be by inhalation, contact, and ingestion. The severity of convulsions and nervous system impairment is dose related. Patients require supportive treatment. Rescuers need SCBA and protective suits (according to the exposure level of the agent).

SAFETY DATA SHEETS (SDSs)

Safety data sheets (SDSs), formerly known as material safety data sheets (MSDSs), explain how to handle caustic substances in the event of an accident or injury and provide pertinent information on the composition and toxic effects of chemicals in a lab. SDSs outline the proper storage of chemicals, procedures for the cleanup and dumping of caustic substances, procedures in the event of a chemical spill or injury, and the proper locations in the facility for cleanup. The SDS should also contain information indicating which substances may cause allergic effects or asthma from contact or inhalation. Emergency rescue services should obtain SDSs for common chemicals and products. Manufacturers and suppliers should have SDSs on file and can be contacted for copies. The OSHA/ Environmental Protection Agency (EPA) Occupational Chemical Database provides links for SDSs for some products. SDSs are available from various other sources, including the Toxicology Data Network (TOXNET) and poison control centers. There are also pathogen safety data sheets for biological hazards.

MULTIPLE-CASUALTY INCIDENTS VERSUS MASS-CASUALTY INCIDENTS

Multiple-casualty incident	Mass-casualty incident
Involves more than one person, but different jurisdictions may quantify the total number of persons differently. Usually refers to an incident involving at least three patients. Usually involves only one jurisdiction and only one to three agencies (ambulance, fire department, and police). Requires triage, but generally only primary. Standards of care are maintained, and all patients not coded black (deceased) are transported for care.	Also involves more than one person, but may involve much larger numbers—dozens, hundreds, to thousands. Often involves multiple jurisdictions and agencies. Requires triage but may also involve separate waiting areas for color-coded individuals and secondary triage. Standards of care may be modified, and patients coded black (expectant) and not expected to live may be left in the field and/or receive delayed care if they are still living after the red- and yellow-coded individuals are transported.

ROLE OF THE TRANSPORTATION OFFICER IN A MASS-CASUALTY INCIDENT

During a mass-casualty event, the **transportation officer** must maintain constant communication with hospitals and trauma centers, triage officers, police, ground ambulance services, and air medical transport services. The transportation officer controls the flow of patients for treatment and must determine where to route patients in order to prevent a backlog at the receiving facility and must coordinate incoming and outgoing ambulances in the transportation staging area. The transportation officer must obtain information about each facility's surge capacity and the number and types of patients the facility is prepared to care for. The transportation officer must also coordinate air medical transport flights and determine, with the triage officer, which patients to transport by air according to their severity of injuries, availability of treatment options, and appropriate levels of care. Speed of transportation and care is often critical in a mass-casualty incident because delays often result in increased death rates.

ROLE OF TRIAGE IN A MASS-CASUALTY INCIDENT RELATED TO TERRORISM OR A DISASTER

In a mass-casualty incident related to terrorism or a disaster, **rapid triage** and tagging must occur and patients must be sorted according to priority for transportation or field treatment. Because of the large numbers of casualties, triage should begin with the first patient encountered, proceeding from one to another. According to some plans, patients who are alive but expected to die are coded red, but this can result in overtriage, with too many red-coded individuals having to be transported and/or treated, resulting in patients dying during the wait. With other plans, patients expected to die are black-coded as "expectant" and left in the field or left aside until red- and yellow-coded individuals are transported and/or treated. If patients are undertriaged (such as patients who should be coded red being coded yellow instead) this can also result in increased deaths while other patients are waiting for transport and/or treatment.

INCREASING SURVIVAL IN MASS-CASUALTY SHOOTING AND IMPROVISED EXPLOSIVE DEVICE INCIDENTS

Terrorist or other attacks that involve active shooters or improvised explosive devices (IEDs) often result in injuries similar to those encountered in combat situations in which the most common causes of death are extremity hemorrhage, tension pneumothorax, and airway obstruction. The **THREAT acronym** provides guidance for dealing with these situations in the following ways:

- Threat suppression: Use of police protection, ballistic vests, concealment, cover, and situational awareness. One concern is that most of the protective gear available to emergency medical personnel is for ballistics rather than explosive devices.
- Hemorrhage control: Use of tourniquets (military style) and hemostatic dressings (QuikClot) to control bleeding.

- Rapid extrication to safety: Move patients and personnel out of the danger zone to prevent further injuries.
- Assessment by medical providers: Includes provision of a nasopharyngeal airway or upright seating and leaning forward for airway compromise and spinal precautions.
- Transport to definitive care: Medical treatment should continue during transport.

SAFETY ISSUES ASSOCIATED WITH ACTIVE SHOOTERS AND TERRORIST BOMB ATTACKS

With **active shooters,** standard protocol has been for emergency response services to wait until the police have removed the threat and secured the area before moving in to care for victims; however, this delay in treatment may result in death, so some authorities are now recommending that emergency response personnel enter the scene with police while wearing appropriate protective equipment, although this does pose some risk, especially with additional shooters or a secondary attack. With a **terrorist bombing** and improvised explosive devices (IEDs), situational awareness is critical because multiple explosive devices (some undetonated) may be at the scene. IEDs may be inside backpacks, suitcases, and packages left unattended, but in emergency situations, innocent people often drop backpacks and packages and run away. Additionally, attackers wearing suicide vests or belts may mix in with other victims or people escaping the blast area.

BOMB THREAT STANDOFF RECOMMENDATIONS

Threat	Explosive capacity (lb)	Mandatory evacuation distance (ft)	Preferred evacuation distance (ft)	Shelter-in-place zone (ft)
Pipe bomb	5	70	1200+	71–1199
Suicide bomber	20	110	1700+	111–1699
Suitcase/Briefcase	50	150	1850+	151–1849
Automobile	500	320	1900+	321–1899
SUV/Van	1000	400	2400+	401–2399
Small truck	4000	640	3800+	641–3799
Container truck	10,000	860	5100+	861–5099
Semitrailer	60,000	1570	9300+	1571–9299

Source: US Department of Homeland Security.

B-NICE HAZARDOUS MATERIAL (HAZMAT) INCIDENTS ASSOCIATED WITH TERRORIST ATTACKS

Category	Response
B—Biological (bacteria, viruses, fungi, toxins)	Inhalation type—evacuate for 80 feet, shut down air-handling systems, wear appropriate PPE and SCBA, and avoid contamination. Visible agent—decontaminate with soap and water. Symptoms may vary but are usually delayed.
N—Nuclear/Radiological	Inhalation type (most common)—Isolate/Secure the area, avoid smoke/fumes, stay upwind, and use PPE and SCBA. Isolate victims and decontaminate as appropriate. Symptoms are usually delayed.
I—Incendiary	Be on alert for multiple devices and sabotaged fire suppression equipment. Symptoms include burns, pain, and trauma.
C—Chemical	Isolate/Secure the area, decontaminate victims with soap and water, and be on alert for chemical dispersal devices. Approach toward uphill and upwind. Isolate symptomatic patients from others. Symptoms vary but may include burns, blistering, vomiting, breathing difficulty, and neurological damage.

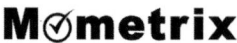

Category	Response
E—Explosives	Be alert for secondary devices, undetonated devices, and secondary hazards (unstable buildings and debris). Remove victims from the area, secure the perimeter, and stage away from the incident area. Decontaminate as necessary. Symptoms include burns, amputations, cuts, and penetrating and blunt trauma.

"ALL-HAZARDS" SAFETY APPROACH TO MASS-CASUALTY INCIDENTS

The **"all-hazards" safety approach** to mass-casualty incidents aims to provide plans that can be used to deal with all types of hazards (natural disasters, terrorist attacks, and mass-casualty incidents) as well as encompassing the four components of emergency management: mitigation, preparedness, response, and recovery. Organizations in an area coordinate to develop joint action plans that can be activated in response to incidents, with the chain of command clearly outlined. This approach lowers costs to individual organizations and provides for faster and more effective response. However, although the basic structure may be the same for responding to all hazards, there are inevitable differences between (for example) a terrorist attack with active shooters and a natural disaster, such as a hurricane, which can be anticipated and mitigated to some degree. For this reason, modifying existing incident action plans to meet the needs of a situation is essential.

TREATING TERRORISTS AND CRIMINALS

In mass-casualty incidents, **terrorists and criminals** involved in the incident may be injured and require treatment, and EMS personnel may feel conflicted about providing treatment when others have been injured or killed, but it's important to provide treatment to terrorists and criminals the same as any other individuals because (1) they are in need of help and (2) their survival may be critical to identifying coconspirators and to providing reasons for the attack. However, these individuals may pose risks to emergency medical personnel, so they should be examined while under police guard. The individual's hands should be examined first to check for weapons and detonators and secured (with handcuffs, if possible). Clothes should be examined and removed very carefully in case the person is wearing a suicide device of some type. Emergency medical personnel should also be aware that the individual may be feigning injury or unconsciousness.

EMT Practice Test

Want to take this practice test in an online interactive format? Check out the online resources page, which includes interactive practice questions and much more: **mometrix.com/resources719/emtint99**

1. All of the following can produce an Antabuse-like reaction except
   a. Antibiotics
   b. Metronidazole
   c. Cocaine
   d. Diabetic medications

2. Lead II on the ECG indicates
   a. Presence of an MI
   b. Regularity of the heartbeat
   c. Pumping capability of the heart
   d. Location of an MI

3. Regular PVCs at intervals greater than every fourth beat are known as
   a. Frequent PVCs
   b. Multifocal PVCs
   c. Ventricular quadrigeminy
   d. Trigeminal PVCs

4. Which of the following statements regarding VT is FALSE?
   a. VT may be associated with cardiac arrest
   b. P waves are usually not discernible
   c. If the rhythm results in a pulse, VT is not significant
   d. Pulseless VT should be treated the same as VF

5. The absence of any electrical activity in the heart is known as
   a. PEA
   b. Asystole
   c. Pericardial tamponade
   d. VF

6. The first step in caring for a patient with cardiac arrest should be to
   a. Set up oxygen and IV lines
   b. Immediately apply the AED
   c. Interpret the patient's cardiac rhythm
   d. Begin CPR

7. All of the following steps in the defibrillation process are valid except
   a. Double-checking the rhythm before delivering a countershock
   b. Turning on the synchronized mode when defibrillating VF
   c. Removing NTG patches before defibrillation
   d. Checking the carotid pulse if the rhythm changes

8. The best line of care for a patient who is hyperventilating is to
    a. Plug the portals of the oxygen mask to induce rebreathing
    b. Ask the patient to breathe into a paper bag
    c. Administer oxygen
    d. Administer a nebulized bronchodilator

9. Spontaneous pneumothorax may be caused by
    a. Smoking
    b. Anxiety
    c. Carbon monoxide
    d. Oral contraceptives

10. Which of the following may be useful in a patient with carbon monoxide poisoning?
    a. Pulse oximetry
    b. Oxygen saturation
    c. Hyperbaric oxygen
    d. Blood glucose

11. All of the following may cause coma except
    a. Vitamin deficiency
    b. Hypercalcemia
    c. Hyperglycemia
    d. Fever

12. A common cause of seizures in adults is
    a. Fever
    b. Infection
    c. Vitamin deficiency
    d. Catatonia

13. Which of the following statements regarding seizure is FALSE?
    a. Seizure patients may bite their tongue
    b. Seizure may result in a neurological condition similar to stroke
    c. Restraining muscle movement may stop a seizure
    d. A patient may become violent after a seizure

14. The roommate of a 21-year-old woman calls you to their apartment. The young woman has severe abdominal pain and vaginal bleeding and has gone into shock. This patient is most likely suffering from
    a. Appendicitis
    b. PID
    c. Bowel obstruction
    d. Ectopic pregnancy

15. The best course of treatment for a patient with hypoglycemia is to give the patient
    a. Saccharine
    b. Aspartame
    c. Oral glucose
    d. Insulin

16. Which of the following conditions is associated with an acetone-like breath odor?
    a. Hypoglycemia
    b. Hyperglycemia
    c. Diabetes
    d. DKA

17. Signs and symptoms of HHNC include
    a. Kussmaul respirations
    b. Fruity breath odor
    c. Altered mental status
    d. Rapid pulse

18. When treating a poisoning victim, which of the following takes LOWEST priority?
    a. Determining the exact substance the patient has taken
    b. Placing the patient on a cardiac monitor
    c. Proper positioning of the patient
    d. Pulse oximetry

19. Proper care for a patient with heat stroke includes
    a. Salt pills
    b. Diuretics
    c. Air conditioning
    d. Cold drinks

20. Which of the following statements regarding hypothermia is FALSE?
    a. Hypothermia may resemble cardiac arrest
    b. Rewarming the extremities may increase body temperature
    c. Hypothermia may mimic death
    d. Rewarming the extremities may decrease body temperature

21. Asthma in children is associated with
    a. Age 6 to 18 months
    b. Viral infection
    c. Family history
    d. Pneumonia

22. In pediatric patients, bronchiolitis is
    a. Seasonal
    b. Caused by a virus
    c. Associated with asthma
    d. Responsive to medication

23. The most important intervention in a child with head trauma is
    a. Immobilization
    b. Ventilation
    c. Resuscitation
    d. Transport

24. The first line of treatment for a child with severe hypothermia should include
    a. Performing CPR
    b. Rubbing the affected extremities
    c. Endotracheal intubation
    d. High-concentration oxygen

25. All of the following may be used in patients with shock except
    a. Lactated Ringer's solution
    b. 5% Dextrose in water
    c. Normal saline
    d. Plasma

26. All of the following are symptoms of cholinergic crisis except
    a. Salivation
    b. Incontinence
    c. Cardiac arrest
    d. Emesis

27. In patient triage, which of the following conditions would be considered high-priority?
    a. Respiratory arrest
    b. Burns
    c. Shock
    d. Spinal cord damage

28. An Apgar score of 10 in a newly born infant indicates
    a. Moderate distress
    b. No distress
    c. Severe distress
    d. Cyanosis

29. The first step in treatment of cardiopulmonary arrest in a newly born infant is
    a. Intubation
    b. IV fluids
    c. Ventilation
    d. Atropine

30. The Apgar score should be obtained
    a. At one and five minutes after birth
    b. Before beginning resuscitation
    c. Immediately at birth
    d. Only if resuscitation is needed

31. The "G" component of the Apgar score stands for
    a. Grimace
    b. Grasp
    c. Good respiratory effort
    d. Growth

32. Which of the following may be administered to a newborn with hypoglycemia and altered consciousness?
    a. 25% dextrose and water
    b. 10% dextrose and water
    c. 50% dextrose and water
    d. Ringer's lactate

33. After an infant's head is delivered, the first line of action should be to
    a. Suction the nose
    b. Suction the mouth
    c. Cover the head
    d. Dry the head

34. Secondary apnea in a newborn is treated by
    a. Touching the infant
    b. Suctioning the mouth
    c. Suctioning the nose
    d. Assisted ventilation

35. Drug withdrawal or overdose may be treated by
    a. Antabuse
    b. Oxygen
    c. Ice immersion
    d. Ipecac

36. All of the following may mimic alcohol intoxication except
    a. Hypoglycemia
    b. Head trauma
    c. Antabuse
    d. Drug abuse

37. In elderly patients, symptoms of which of the following can mimic those of cardiac or respiratory conditions?
    a. Alcohol abuse
    b. Drug abuse
    c. Depression
    d. Psychosis

38. The drug cocaine is classified as a
    a. Hallucinogen
    b. Stimulant
    c. Narcotic
    d. Depressant

39. The suffix "phasia" refers to
    a. Speech
    b. Fear
    c. Order
    d. Eating

40. The prefix "endo" refers to
    a. On
    b. Swelling
    c. Within
    d. Outer

41. Cardiac tamponade typically results from
    a. Head trauma
    b. Bleeding
    c. Cardiac arrest
    d. Chest trauma

42. COPD and respiratory failure may result in
    a. Respiratory alkalosis
    b. Respiratory acidosis
    c. Stroke
    d. Pneumothorax

43. Which of the following drugs is used for patients with acute MI?
    a. Adenosine
    b. Aspirin
    c. Amiodarone
    d. Dexamethasone

44. Vasopressin may be given in all of the following cases except
    a. As an alternative to epinephrine
    b. To treat PEA
    c. To pediatric patients with VF
    d. To treat asystole

45. Epinephrine is contraindicated in
    a. Hypotension
    b. Hypertension
    c. Cardiac arrest
    d. Asthma

46. An area of potential threat in law enforcement operations is known as the
    a. Hot zone
    b. Warm zone
    c. Cold zone
    d. HAZMAT zone

47. A common cause of asymmetric pupils in an elderly patient is
    a. COPD
    b. Skull fracture
    c. CHF
    d. Glaucoma

48. Treatment of a child with hypothermia with a discernible heart rate should include
   a. Tracheal intubation
   b. CPR
   c. Resuscitation
   d. Starting an IV

49. Which of the following statements regarding chest and abdominal trauma in a child is FALSE?
   a. Treatment of chest and abdominal trauma should be the same as that for an adult
   b. Respiratory distress may be a sign of abdominal trauma
   c. The ideal treatment for a child with chest trauma is rapid transport to a hospital
   d. Abdominal trauma should ideally be treated in the field

50. Which of the following is recommended for cervical spine immobilization in a small child?
   a. Using a KED
   b. Using cravats
   c. Strapping the child under the axillae
   d. Pulling the child's head from the safety seat

51. All of the following may be used to treat seizures in a child except
   a. Rectal diazepam
   b. IV glucose
   c. IV lorazepam
   d. IV lactated Ringer's solution

52. Stiffness of the neck and Kernig's sign are symptoms of
   a. Epilepsy
   b. Head trauma
   c. Meningitis
   d. Shock

53. Rales are indicative of which pediatric condition?
   a. Shock
   b. Pneumonia
   c. Bronchiolitis
   d. Croup

54. In a child, shock may be indicated by
   a. Mottling of the skin
   b. Hypertension
   c. Rales
   d. Respiratory distress

55. Which of the following may be used during intraosseous infusion in a child?
   a. Hypodermic needles
   b. Spinal needles
   c. Normal saline
   d. Nasal cannula

56. Compared with adults, which of the following is less likely to be injured in children?
    a. Head
    b. Ribs
    c. Liver
    d. Nerves

57. Which of the following statements regarding a pregnant trauma victim is FALSE?
    a. The heart rate is increased
    b. The BP is lower
    c. The patient should be supine
    d. The patient should be placed on her left side

58. A condition in pregnant women marked by hypertension and fluid retention is known as
    a. Ectopic pregnancy
    b. Gestational diabetes
    c. Preeclampsia
    d. Uterine rupture

59. A typical sign of placenta previa during pregnancy is
    a. Severe abdominal pain
    b. Painless bright red bleeding
    c. Minimal vaginal bleeding
    d. Palpable fetus in abdomen

60. In the case of a prolapsed cord presentation, the EMT-I should
    a. Place the mother in a knee-to-chest position
    b. Push the cord back inside
    c. Form a "V" with the fingers on either side of the infant's nose and mouth
    d. Cut the umbilical cord

61. Which of the following should NOT be used for resuscitation of the newly born?
    a. Atropine
    b. Epinephrine
    c. Dextrose in water
    d. Naloxone

62. Postpartum hemorrhage may be treated by all of the following except
    a. Uterine massage
    b. Fluid bolus
    c. IV line
    d. Trendelenburg positioning

63. Right lower quadrant abdominal pain is usually indicative of
    a. Cirrhosis
    b. Appendicitis
    c. Bowel obstruction
    d. Diverticulitis

64. **Epigastric pain is associated with**
    a. Appendicitis
    b. Ectopic pregnancy
    c. Myocardial ischemia
    d. Hernia

65. **In which of the following cases is NTG contraindicated?**
    a. BP greater than 100 mm Hg
    b. NTG prescription
    c. BP below 100 mm Hg
    d. Headache

66. **Which of the following statements regarding use of NTG is FALSE?**
    a. NTG may be associated with hypotension
    b. NTG tablets may retain potency for months or years
    c. NTG may be associated with headache
    d. NTG tablets may become inactivated by exposure to air or light

67. **Patients with chest pain should be assumed to have**
    a. Angina
    b. Cardiac arrest
    c. Congestive heart failure
    d. MI

68. **Acute MI often presents as**
    a. Indigestion
    b. Nephrolithiasis
    c. Peptic ulcer
    d. Cholecystitis

69. **All of the following are indicative of cardiogenic shock except**
    a. Altered mental status
    b. Hypotension
    c. Peripheral vein collapse
    d. Respiratory distress

70. **Which of the following drugs is contraindicated in pulmonary edema?**
    a. NTG
    b. Morphine
    c. Furosemide
    d. Epinephrine

71. **The signs and symptoms of pulmonary embolism may mimic those of all of the following except**
    a. Pneumonia
    b. MI
    c. CHF
    d. Pneumothorax

72. A barrel-shaped chest is a sign of
    a. Asthma
    b. COPD
    c. Pulmonary embolism
    d. Spontaneous pneumothorax

73. Plasma is also known as
    a. Intracellular fluid
    b. Extracellular fluid
    c. Interstitial fluid
    d. Intravascular fluid

74. Lactated Ringer's solution is a type of
    a. Hypertonic solution
    b. Isotonic solution
    c. Hypotonic solution
    d. Electrolyte

75. Which of the following is an example of a cation?
    a. ATP
    b. Chloride
    c. Sodium
    d. Phosphate

76. The delivery of oxygenated blood to the tissues is known as
    a. Perfusion
    b. Aerobic metabolism
    c. Anaerobic metabolism
    d. Oxygenation

77. Kussmaul breathing is indicative of
    a. Metabolic alkalosis
    b. Metabolic acidosis
    c. Respiratory acidosis
    d. Respiratory alkalosis

78. Shock is typically caused by all of the following except
    a. Fluid loss
    b. Vasodilation
    c. Hypertension
    d. Pump failure

79. Sites in the body where two bones converge are known as
    a. Cartilage
    b. Joints
    c. Tendons
    d. Ligaments

80. An abnormal accumulation of fluid in the pleural cavity is known as
   a. Pneumothorax
   b. Pleural effusion
   c. Respiratory alkalosis
   d. Cardiac tamponade

81. Which of the following components of the APVU mnemonic is incorrect?
   a. A = awake and alert
   b. U = unresponsive
   c. V = vision impaired
   d. P = responsive to painful stimuli

82. The carotid pulse is used to assess the circulation when
   a. The patient is responsive
   b. The patient is unresponsive
   c. The patient is less than 1 year old
   d. The patient is pulseless

83. Which of the following statements regarding baseline vital signs is FALSE?
   a. Vital signs may vary by age
   b. Vital signs should be assessed constantly
   c. Vital signs should be assessed as a set
   d. Vital signs should be assessed individually

84. A normal respiratory rate for an adult would be
   a. 60 times per minute
   b. 40 times per minute
   c. 30 times per minute
   d. 20 times per minute

85. Melena is characterized by
   a. Vomiting of blood
   b. Bright red blood in stool
   c. Black, tarry stool
   d. Acute MI

86. Acute abdomen is caused by all of the following except
   a. Black widow spider bite
   b. Diabetic ketoacidosis
   c. Myocardial infarction
   d. Dog bite

87. Which of the following is a sign of increased heat production?
   a. Sweating
   b. Shivering
   c. Decreased appetite
   d. Decreased voluntary activity

88. All of the following are signs and symptoms of heat stroke except
    a. Altered level of consciousness
    b. Shortness of breath
    c. Profuse sweating
    d. Minimal or no sweating

89. Which of the following is NOT a sign of heat exhaustion?
    a. Profuse sweating
    b. Altered mental status
    c. Pallor
    d. Hypotension

90. In treating a patient with hypothermia, the EMT-I should
    a. Start an IV line with lactated Ringer's solution
    b. Rewarm the extremities
    c. Immerse the patient in warm water
    d. Cover the patient with a blanket

91. Which of the following is associated with the best prognosis?
    a. Dry drowning
    b. Wet drowning
    c. Secondary drowning
    d. Seawater drowning

92. All of the following are used to assess successful ET tube placement in an infant except
    a. Passage of the tube through the vocal cords
    b. Breath sounds
    c. Improvement in color
    d. Rise and fall of the chest

93. Which of the following statements regarding PPE is FALSE?
    a. Prescription glasses with side shields are acceptable eye protection
    b. Surgical masks protect against TB
    c. Coveralls are preferable to gowns as protection against body fluid exposure
    d. Vinyl gloves should never be reused

94. An effective alternative to commercial disinfectants would be
    a. Soap and water
    b. Antiseptics
    c. Bleach and water
    d. Antibacterials

95. Treatment of a severely injured patient who is under arrest would be permissible according to
    a. Implied consent
    b. Involuntary consent
    c. Informed consent
    d. Expressed consent

96. Which of the following statements regarding refusal of care is FALSE?
    a. Mentally incompetent patients cannot give consent
    b. Unemancipated minors cannot refuse care
    c. Emancipated minors can refuse care
    d. Mentally incompetent patients can refuse care

97. All of the following types of patients can be treated under implied consent except
    a. Mentally incompetent adult
    b. Intoxicated adult
    c. Emotionally disturbed minor
    d. Minor when a guardian is unavailable

98. The most common neurotransmitter in the sympathetic nervous system is
    a. Acetylcholine
    b. Norepinephrine
    c. Adrenalin
    d. Epinephrine

99. An example of a parasympathetic response is
    a. Tachycardia
    b. Nervousness
    c. Abdominal distress
    d. Elevated blood pressure

100. Which of the following is almost always indicative of an abnormality?
    a. S_3
    b. S_4
    c. Murmur
    d. SA node

101. Guaifenesin is classified as a _____ drug.
    a. Schedule I
    b. Schedule V
    c. Schedule IV
    d. Schedule II

102. Morphine is an example of a _____ drug.
    a. Schedule II
    b. Schedule I
    c. Schedule IV
    d. Schedule V

103. A drug classified as Pregnancy Category A is considered
    a. Contraindicated in pregnant women
    b. At remote risk of fetal harm
    c. At risk of fetal harm in animals but not humans
    d. Acceptable for use in life-threatening conditions when benefits outweigh risks

104. Acetaminophen concentrations would appear significantly higher in
    a. A 75-year-old obese patient
    b. A 25-year-old obese patient
    c. A 21-year-old normal-weight patient
    d. A 45-year-old slim patient

105. All of the following can be administered in drug form except
    a. Edrophonium
    b. Pilocarpine
    c. Acetylcholine
    d. Atropine

106. An example of a sympathetic agonist drug is
    a. Propranolol
    b. Atropine
    c. Albuterol
    d. Acetylcholine

107. Drugs given by the sublingual route are
    a. Applied directly to the skin
    b. Placed under the tongue
    c. Dissolved between the cheek and gum
    d. Injected into the dermis

108. All of the following drugs can be administered through the endotracheal tube except
    a. Epinephrine
    b. Naloxone
    c. Metaproterenol
    d. Lidocaine

109. The fastest route of drug administration is the _____ route.
    a. Oral
    b. Intravenous
    c. Topical
    d. Endotracheal

110. An acute systemic reaction to a drug on subsequent exposure is known as
    a. Drug toxicity
    b. Tachyphylaxis
    c. Drug dependence
    d. Anaphylaxis

111. An example of drug synergism is
    a. Antacids taken with tetracycline
    b. Sedatives taken with barbiturates
    c. Cimetidine taken with imipramine
    d. Morphine taken with meperidine

112. **All of the following produce a drug interaction except**
    a. Epinephrine taken with digoxin
    b. Phenergan taken with meperidine
    c. Amiodarone taken with digoxin
    d. Methyldopa taken with MAO inhibitors

113. **In a critically injured patient, an IV line should be placed**
    a. En route to the hospital
    b. At the scene before transport
    c. In sclerotic veins
    d. After circulatory collapse

114. **Lactated Ringer's solution contains**
    a. Free water
    b. HCO_3
    c. Calcium
    d. Calories

115. **Which of the following can be administered with blood products?**
    a. Lactated Ringer's solution
    b. Sodium chloride 0.9%
    c. Five percent dextrose in water
    d. Glucose

116. **No restriction of fluid flow from the IV bag to the patient is known as the**
    a. TKO rate
    b. KVO rate
    c. Wide-open rate
    d. Macrodrip

117. **Large-bore catheters should be used for all of the following except**
    a. Administration of 50% dextrose
    b. Administration of blood
    c. Shock patients
    d. Elderly patients

118. **For patient in cardiac arrest, the preferred site for IV cannulation is the**
    a. Jugular vein
    b. Saphenous vein of the leg
    c. Peripheral veins of the antecubital fossa
    d. Peripheral veins of the distal extremities

119. **Use of an armboard may be required in all of the following situations except**
    a. When the antecubital fossa is the venipuncture site
    b. When the wrist is the venipuncture site
    c. In a disoriented or confused patient
    d. In elderly patients

120. Which of the following statements regarding documentation of IV cannulation is FALSE?

   a. Unsuccessful attempts to start the IV must be documented
   b. Tape should be applied over the dressing and then labeled
   c. Tape should be labeled and then applied over the dressing
   d. Type and gauge of the needle should be documented

121. A pyrogenic reaction may result from

   a. Bacteria in the venipuncture site
   b. Air entering the vein
   c. Foreign proteins in the IV solution
   d. Injury to the blood vessel

122. All of the following may be helpful in placing an IV line in a moving patient except

   a. Using an armboard to immobilize extremities
   b. Choosing smaller veins
   c. Choosing the largest vein available
   d. Using a crossover taping technique

123. Which of the following drugs can only be administered by IV push?

   a. Atropine
   b. Epinephrine 1:1000
   c. 1 g/5 mL lidocaine
   d. Adenosine

124. Two syringes are required for preparation of

   a. Ampules
   b. Reconstituted medications
   c. Piggyback infusions
   d. Intradermal TB tests

125. The subcutaneous route is used for administration of all of the following except

   a. Vaccines
   b. Insulin
   c. Lidocaine
   d. Epinephrine

126. Which of the following IM injections sites is not recommended for young children?

   a. Dorsogluteal muscle
   b. Vastus lateralis muscle
   c. Ventrogluteal muscle
   d. Deltoid muscle

127. The needle is injected at a 90-degree angle to the skin in which type of injection?

   a. Intradermal
   b. Intramuscular
   c. Subcutaneous
   d. Endotracheal

128. Medications may be delivered via the pulmonary route through all of the following except
   a. Nebulizer
   b. ET tube
   c. IO infusion
   d. MDI

129. Which of the following statements regarding ET administration is FALSE?
   a. Drug dosages should be 2 to 2.5 times those used for IV or IO administration
   b. Medications must be diluted with normal saline
   c. The needle should be injected through the side of the ET tube
   d. CPR should be stopped during ET administration

130. The space between the lungs is known as the
   a. Thoracic cavity
   b. Mediastinum
   c. Abdominal cavity
   d. Pelvic cavity

131. The number of cervical vertebrae in the neck is
   a. 5
   b. 33
   c. 7
   d. 12

132. How many ribs form the rib cage?
   a. 10 pairs
   b. 12 pairs
   c. 2 pairs
   d. 4 pairs

133. The forearm is composed of which of the following?
   a. Carpals
   b. Metacarpals
   c. Phalanges
   d. Radius

134. Which of the following statements regarding the lymphatic system is FALSE?
   a. Lymph originates from excess cellular fluid
   b. Lymph nodes trap bacteria
   c. Swelling of the lymph nodes indicates dysfunction of the lymphatic system
   d. Swelling of the lymph nodes indicates proper functioning of the lymphatic system

135. In assessing a patient, the resuscitation phase may be performed concurrently with the
   a. Focused history
   b. Initial survey
   c. Physical examination
   d. Rapid trauma assessment

136. During rapid trauma assessment, the EMT-I should assess which part of the body first?
   a. Abdomen
   b. Chest
   c. Lungs
   d. Head

137. All of the following may be used to obtain a more accurate respiratory rate except
   a. Continuing to take the pulse but counting respirations instead
   b. Placing the patient's arm across his or her chest but counting respirations instead
   c. Keeping your hands on the patient but counting respirations instead
   d. Assessing the rise and fall of the patient's chest

138. Absence of breathing is known as
   a. Eupnea
   b. Bradypnea
   c. Apnea
   d. Tachypnea

139. Pulse oximetry is reliable in monitoring arterial oxygen saturation in
   a. Patients in stable condition
   b. Patients in cardiac arrest
   c. Patients with anemia
   d. Patients with hypotension

140. Which of the following statements regarding the detailed assessment is FALSE?
   a. Detailed assessment of a priority patient should be done during transport
   b. A head-to-toe examination is required before transport
   c. An elderly patient should be addressed by his or her formal name
   d. Patient history may be obtained from bystanders

141. All of the following may be indicative of drug use except
   a. Unequal pupils
   b. Dilated pupils
   c. Constricted pupils
   d. Unresponsive pupils

142. Which of the following is symptomatic of subcutaneous emphysema?
   a. Neck vein distention
   b. Battle's sign
   c. Crackling below the skin
   d. Ecchymosis

143. The maximum score on the Glasgow coma scale is
   a. 6
   b. 9
   c. 3
   d. 15

144. Elastic connective tissue covered by mucous membranes that prevents foreign materials from entering the airway is known as the
   a. Glottis
   b. False vocal cords
   c. True vocal cords
   d. Adam's apple

145. Carbon dioxide is carried to the lungs by all of the following means except
   a. In plasma
   b. With hemoglobin
   c. With oxygen
   d. With water

146. With 50% oxygen saturation, the PO$_2$ falls to
   a. 27 mm Hg
   b. 20 mm Hg
   c. 40 mm Hg
   d. 60 mm Hg

147. Upper airway obstruction may be caused by all of the following except
   a. Teeth
   b. Cricoid pressure
   c. Vomiting
   d. Smoke inhalation

148. The whistle-top suctioning catheter is useful in
   a. Removing large volumes of secretions
   b. Removing large food particles
   c. Laryngoscopy
   d. Removing fluids from the lower respiratory tract

149. All of the following are useful in providing assisted breathing except
   a. Demand-valve resuscitator
   b. Whistle-top suctioning catheter
   c. Mouth-to-mouth breathing
   d. Mouth-to-mask breathing

150. The esophageal-tracheal Combitube should be used in
   a. Semiresponsive patients
   b. Patients with esophageal disease
   c. Unconscious patients
   d. Patients with a gag reflex

Answer Key and Explanations

1. C: Some commonly prescribed drugs can produce a reaction similar to that of the drug disulfiram (Antabuse), used in patients with chronic alcohol abuse, following alcohol ingestion; these drugs include metronidazole, antibiotics, and oral diabetic medications.

2. B: Lead II on the ECG is most commonly used for continuous patient monitoring in the prehospital setting and indicates the rate and regularity of the patient's heartbeat; however, it does not indicate the presence or location of a myocardial infarction (MI) or the pumping capability of the heart.

3. A: Regular premature ventricular complexes (PVCs) occurring at intervals greater than every fourth beat are simply called frequent PVCs; a PVC at every fourth beat is known as ventricular quadrigeminy and at every third beat, ventricular trigeminy or a trigeminal PVC. PVCs arising in several areas of the ventricles that differ from each other are known as multifocal PVCs.

4. C: Ventricular tachycardia (VT) is a condition in which three or more PVCs occur in a row; P waves are usually not discernible, and T waves may or may not be present. VT should always be considered significant, even if the rhythm results in a pulse as it may lead to cardiac arrest. Patients with pulseless VT should be treated the same as those with ventricular fibrillation (VF).

5. B: The absence of any electrical activity in the heart is known as asystole. Pulseless electrical activity (PEA) is a condition in which electrical activity in the heart is not properly converted to effective cardiac contraction; pericardial tamponade is a reversible cause of PEA. Ventricular fibrillation (VF) is the erratic firing of multiple sites in the ventricle.

6. D: The first step in caring for a patient with cardiac arrest is to immediately begin CPR. If only one EMT-I is present, he or she should perform CPR according to local protocols and then apply the automated external defibrillator (AED); if two or more EMT-Is are present, one should perform CPR and the other operate the AED. Defibrillation should not be delayed to set up oxygen or IV lines. Because the AED automatically analyzes heart rhythm, it is not necessary for an EMT-I to interpret cardiac rhythms to use an AED.

7. B: When defibrillating a patient with ventricular fibrillation (VF), the EMT-I should ensure that the synchronized mode is turned off. NTG patches should be removed before defibrillation to prevent the patch from exploding and burning the patient. Before delivering a countershock, the EMT-I should double-check the rhythm to ensure that the patient has not reverted to another rhythm. Upon changes in the rhythm or following three sequential shocks, the carotid pulse should be checked.

8. C: When treating hyperventilation, oxygen should be given by nasal cannula. Having the patient breathe into a paper bag or blocking off the portals of an oxygen mask to induce rebreathing is no longer considered acceptable practice as it may lead to hypoxia. Nebulized bronchodilators are used to treat acute chronic obstructive pulmonary disease (COPD).

9. A: Spontaneous pneumothorax, or the sudden collapse of the lung, is associated with a variety of risk factors including smoking, COPD, lower respiratory infection, and activities associated with pressure changes, such as scuba diving. Anxiety may result in hyperventilation, particular episodes of anxiety attacks. Oral contraceptives have a known risk factor for causing deep venous thrombosis. Carbon monoxide poisoning causes headache, dizziness, weakness, mental status changes, and nausea/vomiting.

10. C: In the case of carbon monoxide poisoning, pulse oximetry and oxygen saturation readings may be inaccurate; hyperbaric oxygen may be useful if the patient is unresponsive, combative, or hallucinating. Measuring the blood glucose level may be useful in stroke patients.

11. D: Coma may result from intracranial causes, such as intracranial bleeding, stroke, and infection or from causes outside of the nervous system, such as vitamin deficiency, hyper- or hyponatremia, hypercalcemia, and hyper- or hypoglycemia. Fever may induce seizures in children, and rarely, in adults.

12. B: In adults, seizures may be caused by infections (such as meningitis or encephalitis), trauma, metabolic abnormalities (such as hypercalcemia and hypoglycemia), and liver or kidney failure. Febrile convulsions may cause seizures in children; however, fever is rarely the cause of seizures in adults. Psychiatric conditions such as catatonia may result in coma.

13. C: Restraining a patient during a seizure is not effective in stopping the seizure; placing a pillow or rolled blanket under the patient's head may help prevent injury. During a seizure, patients may bite their mouth or tongue. Following a seizure, patients may become violent. In some patients, a condition may develop that resembles the paralysis experienced by stroke victims; however, the paralysis only lasts for one to two hours.

14. D: Vaginal bleeding and severe abdominal pain in a woman of child-bearing age is most probably due to a ruptured ectopic pregnancy. Appendicitis is associated with right lower quadrant abdominal pain and bowel obstruction with abdominal distention; pelvic inflammatory disease (PID) is inflammation of the female internal genitalia due to sexually transmitted disease and is marked by lower abdominal pain, vaginal discharge, fever, and chills.

15. C: For a patient with hypoglycemia, the best course of treatment is to give the patient oral glucose or sugar; sugar substitutes such as saccharine or aspartame are not effective because they do not contain sugar. Insulin should never be given to a patient who may be diabetic.

16. D: Diabetic ketoacidosis (DKA) is associated with a fruity, acetone-like odor of the breath; however, this does not occur in all patients with DKA.

17. C: Hyperosmolar hyperglycemic nonketotic coma (HHNC) typically occurs in patients older than 60 years living in a nursing home or institutional setting and may result from infection, extreme cold, or dehydration. HHNC is usually associated with gradual deterioration of mental status. Kussmaul respirations and fruity breath odor are associated with DKA and are absent in patients with HHNC.

18. A: In treating a patient who has ingested poison, it is not necessary for the EMT-I to determine the exact substance the patient has taken. The airway should be maintained and pulse oximetry monitored; the patient should be placed on a cardiac monitor and positioned in the left lateral recumbent position to prevent aspiration.

19. C: In caring for a patient with heat stroke, placing the patient in a cool environment, such as an air-conditioned ambulance, as soon as possible is vital to prevent brain damage. Salt pills or cold, salty, or sweet drinks should not be given to prevent nausea and vomiting. Heat exhaustion commonly occurs in patients taking diuretics.

20. B: Severe hypothermia may mimic cardiac arrest or clinical death. In treating a patient with hypothermia, rewarming of the extremities may actually decrease body temperature and lead to shock.

21. C: In pediatric patients, asthma can occur at any age and may be a response to allergy or exercise; most pediatric asthma patients have a family history of asthma. Viral infection is associated with bronchiolitis. Pneumonia is an infection of the lower airway or lung caused by a bacteria or virus.

22. B: In pediatric patients, bronchiolitis is an infection of the lower respiratory tract caused by a virus; it may occur at any time and is not associated with a history of asthma. Bronchiolitis is often unresponsive to medication.

23. B: The most important intervention in a child with head trauma is ventilation by either bag-valve-mask device or endotracheal intubation to prevent further injury and sustain neurologic function.

24. D: The first priority in treating a child with severe hypothermia is to maintain the airway by providing high-concentration oxygen. Stimulation, including endotracheal intubation, CPR, or suctioning, should be avoided to prevent ventricular fibrillation; rubbing the affected extremities can cause further tissue damage.

25. B: Normal saline and lactated Ringer's solution may be used in patients with shock; however, 5% dextrose in water is not recommended. Plasma may be given in the hospital setting.

26. C: The acronym SLUDGE may be used as a mnemonic device for the symptoms of cholinergic crisis: Salivation, Lacrimation, Urinary incontinence, Defecation (or fecal incontinence), Generalized weakness, and Emesis.

27. C: According to proper triage methods, a patient with signs and symptoms of shock would be considered highest priority; those with burns but without airway compromise or with back injuries with or without spinal cord damage would be considered second priority. A patient in respiratory or cardiopulmonary arrest would be considered lowest priority.

28. B: An Apgar score of 7 to 10 in a newly born infant indicates mild or no distress; a score of 4 to 6 indicates moderate distress, such as cyanosis, and a score of 0 to 3 indicates severe distress.

29. C: The first step in treatment of cardiopulmonary arrest in a newly born infant is to provide ventilation and oxygenation. If the problem does not resolve, intubation, IV fluids, and medications such as atropine, epinephrine, lidocaine, or naloxone should be administered.

30. A: The Apgar score should be obtained in a newly born infant at 1 minute after birth and again at 5 minutes after birth. Waiting to obtain the Apgar score before beginning resuscitation may have disastrous consequences.

31. A: The components of the Apgar score are as follows: A indicates appearance or color; P, pulse or heart rate; G, grimace or irritability; A, activity or muscle tone; and R, respirations.

32. B: Only 10% dextrose and water can be safely given to a newborn infant with hypoglycemia and altered consciousness; hyperosmotic agents such as 25% dextrose and water or 50% dextrose and water may cause hemorrhage. Ringer's lactate is used in the treatment of hypovolemia.

33. B: Immediately after the infant's head is delivered, suction the mouth and then the nose to stimulate breathing. The infant's head, face, and body should then be dried; after this, the head should be covered with a blanket, towel, or hat to prevent heat loss.

34. D: Primary apnea occurs when a newborn is not visibly breathing and may be reversed by touching and stimulating the infant and/or suctioning. Secondary apnea occurs if oxygen deprivation continues; secondary apnea cannot be reversed by stimulation or suctioning and may require assisted ventilation, including bag-mask ventilation with high-concentration oxygen.

35. B: In the case of drug withdrawal or overdose, maintain the airway and monitor the patient's respiratory status; oxygen may be given by nasal cannula or nonbreather mask as per local protocol. Ipecac is seldom prescribed for use in the field and has largely been replaced by activated charcoal and gastric lavage, usually in the hospital. Ice immersion is a form of street treatment and is ineffective. Antabuse, or disulfiram, is a medication taken by patients with chronic alcohol abuse.

36. C: Drug abuse, head trauma, and medical conditions such as hypoglycemia and diabetic ketoacidosis may mimic alcohol intoxication; Antabuse, or disulfiram, is a medication prescribed for patients with chronic alcohol abuse.

37. C: In elderly patients, depression can present as organic illness, such as cardiac or respiratory disease.

38. B: Cocaine is the most widely abused stimulant drug; heroin, morphine, and hydrocodone (Vicodin) are classified as narcotics. LSD, PCP, and mescaline are common hallucinogens; marijuana and barbiturates are common depressants.

39. A: The suffix "phasia" refers to speech; thus, the term aphasia means inability to speak.

40. C: The prefix "endo" refers to within or inner; thus, the term endometrium means within the uterus.

41. D: Cardiac tamponade is associated with penetrating chest trauma in which the pericardial sac fills with fluid, resulting in the signs and symptoms of shock.

42. B: COPD and respiratory failure may block the ability of the lungs to blow off carbon dioxide, causing a build-up of acid in the blood; this condition is referred to as respiratory acidosis. Respiratory alkalosis results from a deficit of carbon dioxide due to hyperventilation, making the blood more alkaline or basic.

43. B: Aspirin is indicated for patients with acute myocardial infarction. Adensosine is indicated for supraventricular tachycardia (SVT) and paroxysmal SVT (PSVT); amiodarone is indicated for ventricular fibrillation (VF) and ventricular tachycardia (VT) and dexamethasone for shock and various inflammatory and allergic disorders.

44. C: Children and geriatric patients have an increased sensitivity to vasopressin; thus, vasopressin is contraindicated in these patients. Vasopressin is indicated as an alternative to the first or second dose of epinephrine for the treatment of shock-refractory ventricular fibrillation (VF), asystole, or pulseless electrical activity (PEA).

45. B: Epinephrine is contraindicated in patients with hypertension, hypothermia, and pulmonary edema; it is indicated in cardiac arrest and asthma.

46. B: During law enforcement operations, the area of immediate or direct threat is known as the hot zone or kill zone; an area of potential threat is known as the warm zone, and an area posing no threat is known as the cold zone.

47. D: Asymmetric pupils in an elderly patient may result from glaucoma or other ocular diseases or from cataract surgery.

48. C: In treating a child with hypothermia, if a heart rate is present, any form of stimulation, including tracheal intubation, CPR, or suctioning, should be avoided to prevent ventricular fibrillation. Resuscitation should continue until the child's temperature returns to normal.

49. D: A child with chest or abdominal trauma should ideally be treated in the same manner as an adult; that is, by rapid transport to a hospital. In the case of a child with suspected abdominal trauma, treatment in the field may result in decompensation. Respiratory distress may be a sign of abdominal trauma.

50. B: An adult vest device such as the Kendrick extrication device (KED) is not recommended for cervical spine immobilization in a small child; placing large, wide straps under the axillae can inhibit brachial circulation. If it is necessary to remove the child from a child safety seat, the child should be moved as a unit; pulling on the head or neck can cause additional injury. Because abdominal excursion is a necessary part of ventilation in a child less than 7 years of age, cravats are preferable to straps.

51. D: Treatment of seizures in a child may include IV diazepam or lorazepam; rectal diazepam is available in a gel and may be easier to use than the IV form. IV glucose may be needed to correct hypoglycemia due to prolonged seizure activity. IV lactated Ringer's solution is used to treat shock in a child with meningitis.

52. C: The presence of neck stiffness and Kernig's sign, or pain on leg extension, is symptomatic of meningitis.

53. B: Rales are indicative of pneumonia in children older than 1 year.

54. A: Because a child's skin is thinner than that of an adult, changes in color or temperature such as mottling may indicate shock; the presence of two different skin colors is common in children in shock.

55. C: Intraosseous infusion is performed in children in severe shock or cardiac arrest; during the procedure, IV fluids such as lactated Ringer's solution or normal saline should be given. Hypodermic needles or spinal needles are not recommended.

56. B: Compared with those of adults, a child's ribs are more pliable and can withstand more force; however, in children, the head is larger and heavier and is more likely to be injured. In children, the internal organs are larger in proportion to body size and the skeletal structure is smaller; thus, children are more prone to internal injuries. The organ most likely to be injured is the liver. Children have immature nervous systems and the nerves are not well insulated.

57. C: In pregnant women, the heart rate is increased, and the blood pressure (BP) is lower. A pregnant patient should be positioned on her left side rather than in the supine position.

58. C: Preeclampsia is a condition occurring in pregnant women marked by hypertension and fluid retention; ectopic pregnancy refers to pregnancy outside the uterus and is characterized by significant vaginal bleeding, abdominal pain, hypotension, and shock. Gestational diabetes may occur in women with preexisting diabetes but may also occur in women who are not diabetic; this condition results in high blood sugar levels and may be treated with diet and exercise. Uterine rupture most commonly occurs after the onset of labor and is marked by severe abdominal pain and a tearing sensation in the abdomen.

59. B: Placenta previa is the abnormal positioning of the placenta within the uterus and is characterized by painless bright red bleeding. Abruptio placentae, also called placenta abruptio, is the premature detachment of the placenta and is characterized by severe abdominal pain, minimal vaginal bleeding, and a palpable fetus in the abdomen.

60. A: In the case of a prolapsed umbilical cord in which the cord presents first during delivery, the mother should be placed in a knee-to-chest or head-and-torso-down position; the cord should never be pushed back inside or cut. In the case of a breech presentation, the EMT-I should form a "V" with his or her fingers on either side of the infant's nose and mouth, and gently guide the head out by lifting the body in a slight anterior position.

61. C: When ventilation and oxygenation are not sufficient in resuscitating a newly born infant, IV fluids and medications such as atropine, epinephrine, naloxone, or lidocaine may be given; dextrose in water is not indicated in resuscitation of the newborn.

62. D: Postpartum hemorrhage may result from vaginal or cervical tearing, bleeding or clotting disorders, or a retained placenta and should be treated with uterine massage; a second IV line may also be started and a fluid bolus administered. Positioning the mother in the knee-to-chest or Trendelenburg position is useful for a prolapsed cord presentation.

63. B: Right lower quadrant abdominal pain is usually indicative of appendicitis unless proven otherwise; symptoms of bowel obstruction include abdominal distention and tenderness. Diverticulitis is characterized by left lower quadrant pain; in cirrhosis, severe abdominal pain may be associated with infected peritoneal fluid.

64. C: Epigastric pain is associated with gastritis, esophagitis, pancreatitis, cholecystitis, abdominal aortic aneurysm, and myocardial ischemia; appendicitis is associated with right lower quadrant pain and hernia with right or left lower quadrant pain. A ruptured ectopic pregnancy is associated with left lower quadrant pain.

65. C: Nitroglycerin (NTG) is contraindicated in patients with systolic BP less than 100 mm Hg, in patients with head injury, and in infants and children; typically, the EMT-I can assist a patient with a prescription for NTG and a systolic BP greater than 100 mm Hg in administering a sublingual tablet or spray. NTG administration may be associated with headache; however, headache is not a contraindication for use of NTG.

66. B: Nitroglycerin (NTG) tablets or spray have an expiration date and may lose potency after exposure to air or light. NTG use may be associated with headache or hypotension.

67. D: Because it is difficult to distinguish acute myocardial infarction (MI) from angina, a patient with chest pain should be assumed to have MI. Cardiac arrest and congestive heart failure are complications of MI.

68. A: Acute MI often presents as epigastric pain; some patients, particularly the elderly, complain of indigestion rather than chest pain.

69. B: Hypotension is not necessarily indicative of cardiogenic shock; patients with preexisting hypertension may have nearly normal blood pressure. Signs and symptoms of cardiogenic shock include altered mental status, collapse of peripheral veins, and respiratory distress.

70. D: Nitroglycerin (NTG), furosemide, and morphine sulfate are indicated for use in patients with pulmonary edema; however, epinephrine is contraindicated.

71. C: Pulmonary embolism may be associated with pleuritic chest pain, respiratory distress, and shortness of breath; signs and symptoms are similar to those of pneumonia, myocardial infarction (MI), and spontaneous pneumothorax.

72. B: A barrel-shaped chest is a sign of chronic obstructive pulmonary disease (COPD).

73. D: Plasma is also known as intravascular fluid; this component of the blood is noncellular and is found within the blood vessels. Intracellular fluid is found within individual cells and extravascular fluid outside of cell membranes; interstitial fluid is located outside of the blood vessels in the spaces between the cells.

74. B: Isotonic solutions have an osmotic pressure equal to normal body fluid; lactated Ringer's solution and 0.9% normal saline are examples of isotonic solutions. Hypotonic solutions have an osmotic pressure less than that of normal body fluids, and hypertonic solutions have an osmotic pressure greater than that of normal fluids. Electrolytes are salts that break into ions when dissolved in a solvent.

75. C: Anions and cations are two types of electrolytes; anions have a negative charge and cations a positive charge. Examples of cations include sodium, potassium, calcium, and magnesium; examples of anions include chloride, phosphate, and bicarbonate. Adenosine triphosphate (ATP) is a chemical substance produced in the mitochondria.

76. A: The delivery of oxygenated blood to the tissues is known as perfusion. Aerobic metabolism allows the body to use food for energy and involves a combination of oxygen and glucose; anaerobic metabolism is metabolism without oxygen and is experienced by patients in shock.

77. B: Kussmaul breathing, or deep, rapid respirations, is indicative of metabolic acidosis, a condition in which bicarbonate levels are low in relation to carbonic acid levels. In metabolic alkalosis, bicarbonate levels are higher than carbonic acid levels; symptoms include slow, shallow respirations. Respiratory acidosis occurs when exhalation of carbon dioxide is inhibited, and respiratory alkalosis occurs when carbon dioxide exhalation is excessive.

78. C: The primary mechanisms of shock are fluid loss, significant vasodilation, and pump failure.

79. B: A joint is a site in the body where two or more bones converge; cartilage is connective tissue that enables bones to move freely. Fibrous tissues that attach muscles to bones are known as tendons; ligaments are a type of fibrous tissue that connects bones or cartilage.

80. B: An abnormal accumulation of fluid in the pleural cavity is known as pleural effusion; a collection of air in the pleural cavity is known as pneumothorax. Respiratory alkalosis is a condition in which a deficit of carbon dioxide causes the blood to become more alkaline. Cardiac tamponade is associated with chest trauma and results when the pericardial sac fills too rapidly with blood, preventing the heart from filling adequately and inducing shock.

81. C: The APVU mnemonic is used to determine the level of the patient's responsiveness to stimuli. A = awake and alert, P = responsive to painful stimuli, V = responsive to verbal stimuli, and U = unresponsive.

82. B: If the patient is responsive, the radial pulse should be checked; however, in unresponsive patients, the carotid pulse should be checked first. In children less than 1 year of age, the brachial or femoral pulse should be palpated.

83. D: No one vital sign can provide adequate information about a patient's condition; thus, vital signs should be assessed as a set. Vital signs can vary widely among individuals and may vary by age; vital signs should be assessed constantly to evaluate changes in the patient's condition.

84. D: The normal respiratory rate for an adult is 12 to 20 times per minute. Newborns breathe at a rate of 40 to 60 times per minute; children 1 year of age breathe 30 to 40 times per minute, and children 3 years of age breathe 25 to 30 times per minute.

85. C: Melena is the presence of black, tarry stool caused by the passing of digested blood through the gastrointestinal tract; hematochezia is the presence of bright red blood in the stool. Hematemesis is the vomiting of blood and is characterized by vomitus with a coffee ground-like appearance due to the digestion of blood by the stomach acid.

86. D: Acute abdomen is the presence of acute abdominal pain not caused by injury and may result from a variety of illnesses not necessarily originating within the abdominal cavity, such as myocardial infarction and diabetic ketoacidosis. Acute abdomen may also be caused by a black widow spider bite; however, it is not associated with a dog bite.

87. B: Shivering is a sign of increased heat production; sweating is a sign of increased heat loss associated with hyperthermic compensation. Decreased appetite and decreased voluntary activity are signs of decreased heat production.

88. C: Signs and symptoms of heat stroke include altered level of consciousness, shortness of breath, and minimal or no sweating.

89. B: Altered mental status is associated with heat stroke and is rarely seen in patients with heat exhaustion. Signs and symptoms of heat exhaustion include profuse sweating, pallor, and hypotension.

90. D: The first step in treating a patient with hypothermia is to remove the patient from the cold environment; if wet, the patient should be dried as much as possible and covered with a blanket, insulating material, and moisture barriers and transported to a warm environment. The EMT-I should not attempt to rewarm the extremities as this may lead to vasodilation of the arms and legs. Warmed IV fluids may be helpful; however, lactated Ringer's solution should not be given because the liver may not be able to metabolize the lactate. Warm water immersion is not useful in the pre-hospital setting.

91. A: In victims of dry drowning, anoxia results from laryngeal spasm, which prevents the entrance of both water and air into the lungs. Dry drowning may result in cerebral anoxia, edema, and unconsciousness;

however, victims of dry drowning have the best chance of survival. In wet drowning, the victim exerts a violent respiratory effort, filling the lungs with water; secondary drowning is the recurrence of respiratory distress after recovery from the initial drowning episode. In victims of seawater drowning, the presence of seawater in the lungs results in an influx of hypotonic serum, leading to profound hypoxemia.

92. B: The definitive method for assessing successful endotracheal (ET) tube placement in an infant is watching the passage of the tube through the vocal cords; breath sounds alone may not indicate successful placement, as sounds are easily transmitted due to the small size of the infant's chest. Improvement in color and heart rate and the rise and fall of the chest indicate successful placement.

93. B: Surgical masks do not provide adequate protection against some airborne pathogens, such as those causing tuberculosis (TB). Although goggles provide the best protection against bloodborne pathogens, prescription glasses with side shields are acceptable. Because coveralls are closer-fitting than gowns, overall-type coveralls with approved barrier shielding are preferable to gowns as protection against exposure to body fluids. Latex or rubber gloves should never be reused.

94. C: Bleach solution diluted in water is an effective alternative to commercial disinfectants. Antiseptics destroy germs on living tissue rather than on nonliving objects; soap and water and antibacterials are not effective alternatives to disinfectants.

95. B: Involuntary consent involves treatment of a patient granted under authority of law whether or not the patient agrees to treatment, This may apply to a patient held for mental health evaluation or a patient who is under arrest; implied consent involves treatment of a patient who is severely ill or injured under the assumption that the patient would want care if able to respond. In the case of expressed consent, the patient gives verbal or written permission to be treated; in the case of informed consent, the patient gives consent to be treated only after receiving all information needed to understand his or her condition.

96. D: An adult who has been legally determined mentally incompetent cannot give consent for or refuse care. In this case, consent is usually given by a legal guardian; however, if the guardian is not available, the patient may receive care under implied consent. Unemancipated minors, or patients younger than 18 years of age, are not able to give or withhold consent; however, emancipated minors who have been legally absolved from the need for parental consent, such as those who are married, parents, or in the armed forces, can give their own consent.

97. C: In most states, minors, or patients under the age of 18 years, cannot legally consent to or refuse care; however, if a parent or guardian is not available, minors can be treated under implied consent. Adults who have been legally declared mentally incompetent can also receive care if a legal guardian is not available; however, adults experiencing alcohol or substance intoxication, emotional or psychiatric problems, or other medical conditions that may temporarily impair the ability to make rational decisions may be treated under implied consent.

98. B: Norepinephrine is the most common neurotransmitter in the sympathetic nervous system; norepinephrine is related to epinephrine or adrenaline, which also functions as a sympathetic neurotransmitter. Acetylcholine is the most common neurotransmitter in the parasympathetic nervous system.

99. C: The parasympathetic nervous system controls intestinal activity, respiratory rate, and pupillary response; examples of a parasympathetic response include abdominal distress and nausea and vomiting. The sympathetic nervous system controls the fight or flight response and causes constriction of blood vessels and elevation of heart rate and blood pressure; sympathetic responses include nervousness and tachycardia.

100. B: The third (S_3) and fourth (S_4) heart sounds are not typically heard in normal individuals; however, while S_3 is sometimes heard in healthy young people, S_4 is almost always indicative of an abnormality. A murmur is an abnormal whooshing sound indicating turbulent blood flow. Many heart murmurs are benign and disappear over time. The SA, or sinoatrial, node is a normal component of the circulatory system.

101. B: Guaifenesin, an ingredient in many cough medicines, is classified as a Schedule V drug, with the lowest potential for abuse; Schedule I drugs have the highest potential for abuse and include heroin, LSD, and mescaline.

102. A: Morphine, codeine, cocaine, and amphetamines are examples of Schedule II drugs with a high potential for abuse; Schedule I drugs, such as heroin, LSD, peyote, and mescaline, have the highest potential for abuse and no accepted medical use in the United States. Schedule V drugs, including guaifenesin and difenoxin/atropine sulfate, have the lowest potential for abuse.

103. B: A drug classified as a Pregnancy Category A drug carries only a remote risk of fetal harm; drugs in Pregnancy Category X are contraindicated in pregnant women. Drugs in Category C have shown evidence of fetal harm in animal but not in human studies; drugs designated Pregnancy Category D may be used to treat life-threatening conditions when the potential benefits of the drug outweigh the risks.

104. A: Certain drugs, such as acetaminophen, morphine, or meperidine, are affected by body weight and appear in significantly higher concentrations in elderly and obese patients than in younger or slim patients; thus, dosage modifications are necessary in elderly or obese patients to prevent overdose.

105. C: Acetylcholine cannot be administered as a drug because it is broken down by cholinesterase in the blood and synapses before it can occupy receptors; however, some drugs, such as pilocarpine, which is used to treat glaucoma, mimic the action of acetylcholine. Edrophonium is a cholinesterase inhibitor; atropine is used to treat cardiovascular conditions.

106. C: Sympathetic agonists affect the alpha- and beta-adrenergic receptors; the asthma drugs albuterol and metaproterenol are known as beta-2 agonists. Propranolol is a common beta blocker. Acetylcholine affects the parasympathetic division but cannot be given as a drug because it is broken down by cholinesterase in the blood and synapses before it can reach the receptors; atropine is an acetylcholine antagonist.

107. B: A drug given by the sublingual route is placed under the tongue; drugs given via the buccal route are dissolved between the cheek and gum. Topical or transdermal medications are applied directly to the skin. Intradermal administration is injection of the drug into the dermis.

108. C: Five drugs can be administered through the endotracheal tube: atropine, epinephrine, lidocaine, naloxone, and vasopressin; metaproterenol is a bronchodilator and is administered via a nebulizer or metered dose inhaler.

109. B: The intravenous route is the fastest route of drug administration while the oral route is the slowest. Drugs administered via the endotracheal route are absorbed rapidly but not immediately. The topical route has a moderate rate of absorption.

110. D: An acute systemic reaction to a drug on subsequent exposure is known as anaphylaxis; anaphylaxis occurs when an individual becomes sensitized to the drug and experiences a sudden, severe whole-body allergic reaction. Tachyphylaxis is the rapid development of tolerance to a drug. Drug dependence is the development of a physical or psychological need to use a drug; drug toxicity results from overdosage, ingestion of a drug meant for external use, or the buildup of a drug concentration in the blood resulting from impaired metabolism or excretion.

111. B: Synergism occurs when two drugs work together to produce an effect neither drug can produce alone; for example, sedatives taken with barbiturates can cause central nervous system depression. Antagonism occurs when one drug prevents the absorption of another drug; for example, antacids taken with tetracycline block the absorption of tetracycline. Potentiation occurs when one drug multiplies the effect of another;

cimetidine taken with imipramine increases the blood levels of imipramine. Meperidine and morphine are both members of the opiate class of drugs.

112. B: Phenergan, a nonnarcotic emetic, and meperidine, a synthetic narcotic analgesic, have a synergistic effect when taken together; that is, both drugs taken together are more effective for pain relief than either drug alone. Epinephrine taken with digoxin produces a drug interaction that increases the risk of cardiac dysrhythmias. When amiodarone,is taken with digoxin, it increases serum digoxin levels, resulting in drug toxicity. Methyldopa taken with monoamine oxidase (MAO) inhibitors may lead to hypertension.

113. A: In a critically injured patient, the EMT-I should not delay transport to the hospital by attempting to start an IV line on the scene; rather, the IV should be started en route to the hospital. An IV line should not be started in sclerotic veins or after the patient experiences circulatory collapse.

114. C: Lactated Ringer's solution contains sodium, potassium, calcium, chloride, and lactate but not HCO_3; it does not provide free water or calories.

115. B: Sodium chloride 0.9% is the only IV solution that can be given with blood products.

116. C: No restriction of fluid flow from the IV bag to the patient is known as the wide-open rate. The TKO, or "to keep open" rate, is equal to approximately 8 to 15 drops of fluid per minute; it is also known as the KVO, or "keep vein open" rate. The macrodrip is a drip chamber used when a large amount of fluid is needed.

117. D: Large-bore, or 14- to 16-guage catheters, may be used for administration of viscous fluids, such as blood or blood components, or viscous medications, such as 50% dextrose. Large-bore catheters should be used for patients in shock, cardiac arrest, or other life-threatening conditions; however, they are not indicated for patients with small or fragile veins, such as infants and children or the elderly.

118. C: In patients in cardiac arrest, the preferred site for IV cannulation is the peripheral veins of the antecubital fossa (the area anterior to and below the elbow); distal peripheral veins are the least preferred site because blood flow from distal extremities is diminished during circulatory collapse. Use of the jugular vein is sometimes contraindicated by local protocols because the catheter and tubing are difficult to tape down and may be easily displaced. The saphenous vein of the leg should only be used as a last resort because of the risk of thrombus formation.

119. D: Use of an armboard may be necessary when the venipuncture device is inserted near a joint, such as in the antecubital fossa or in the dorsum of the hand or wrist. It may also be used with restraints in disoriented or confused patients. Use of the armboard is usually not necessary in noncritical patients.

120. B: In documenting IV placement, the EMT-I should place a piece of tape on a flat surface, write the information on the tape, and then place it directly over the dressing; the tape should not be labeled after it has been applied over the dressing as this may irritate the venipuncture site. Information that should be documented includes the initials of the individual who placed the IV, the date and time of insertion, and the type and gauge of the needle as well as all unsuccessful attempts to start the IV.

121. C: A pyrogenic reaction occurs when foreign proteins capable of producing a fever are present in the administration set or the IV solution. A hematoma may result from injury to a blood vessel; a local infection may occur when appropriate cleansing techniques have not been used and bacteria enter the venipuncture site. An air embolism occurs when air enters the vein.

122. B: In placing an IV line in a patient who is moving or having a seizure, the extremity should be held as still as possible; an armboard may be useful to immobilize the extremity and prevent accidental displacement of the cannula. Choose the largest vein available; using smaller veins increases the risk of the needle passing through the vein in the event of sudden movement. Using a crossover taping technique is acceptable to prevent the catheter from being dislodged from the vein.

123. D: Adenosine, an atrial antidysrhythmic, can only be given by IV push, whereas atropine, a parasympatholytic, can be given endotracheally, intramuscularly, or by IV push. Epinephrine in a 1:1000 concentration can be given subcutaneously, whereas epinephrine in a 1:10,000 concentration may be administered either endotracheally or by IV push. Administration of 1g/5 mL lidocaine by IV push may result in severe adverse events.

124. B: Two syringes are required for preparation of reconstituted medications; the first syringe is used to add the sterile liquid and the second to inject the medication after it has been mixed. Ampules are breakable glass containers from which drugs are drawn with a syringe. Attaching a continuous infusion to a primary IV line is known as a piggyback infusion. Intradermal tuberculin (TB) skin tests are administered using a TB syringe.

125. C: The subcutaneous route is used for the administration of epinephrine, insulin, heparin, and some vaccines; lidocaine is administered by the IV route.

126. A: The dorsogluteal injection site is not recommended for children under the age of 3 years because the muscle is not yet developed and injection at this site may result in penetration of the sciatic nerve. The vastus lateralis muscle is the preferred site for injection in children less than 3 years of age; the ventrogluteal and deltoid muscles may be used for young children.

127. B: When administering an intramuscular injection, the needle is injected at a 90-degree angle to the skin; with an intradermal injection, the angle of the needle is 15 degrees and with a subcutaneous injection, 45 degrees. In endotracheal administration, drugs are introduced directly through the endotracheal tube in an intubated patient.

128. C: Medications may be administered as an aerosol via the pulmonary route using a nebulizer, metered dose inhaler (MDI), or endotracheal (ET) tube; intraosseous (IO) infusion is the infusion of fluid or medication directly into the bone marrow.

129. C: Drug levels achieved through endotracheal (ET) administration are less than those achieved through the IV or intraosseous (IO) routes; thus, drug dosages should be 2 to 2.5 times the recommended dose for IV or IO administration. Medications must be diluted with normal saline before ET administration. The needle should not be injected through the side of the ET tube for medication delivery. If CPR is being delivered at the same time as ET drug injection, chest compressions should be stopped temporarily until several ventilations are given.

130. B: The space between the lungs is known as the mediastinum; the thoracic cavity is located between the base of the neck and the diaphragm and is formed by the boundary of the rib cage. The abdominal cavity extends from the diaphragm to the pelvic bones and comprises the gastrointestinal and urinary systems. The pelvic cavity comprises the lower portion of the abdominal cavity and is bordered by the pelvic bones.

131. C: The spine consists of 33 bones called vertebrae and is divided into 5 sections; there are 7 cervical vertebrae in the neck. There are 12 thoracic vertebrae in the posterior chest.

132. B: A total of 12 pairs of ribs form the rib cage; the upper 10 attach directly to the sternum and the remaining 2 pairs are held together by cartilage. Four vertebrae are fused into the coccyx or tailbone.

133. D: The forearm is composed of two bones: the radius and the ulna. The carpals comprise the wrist and the metacarpals form the hand. The phalanges are the small bones that comprise the fingers.

134. C: Lymph originates from excess cellular fluid and circulates throughout the body in lymph vessels; lymphatic fluid is filtered in the lymph nodes and travels back to the circulatory system via the thoracic duct. Bacteria and viruses are trapped in the lymph nodes until they are destroyed by the immune system; thus, swelling of the lymph nodes during an infection indicates that the lymphatic system is functioning properly.

135. B: In the resuscitation phase, life-saving procedures such as relief of airway obstruction, CPR, and control of hemorrhage should be performed. The resuscitation phase may be performed concurrently with the initial survey; if a life-threatening condition is detected during the initial survey, the survey should be stopped and the condition treated before continuing the survey. The EMT-I should reconsider the mechanism of injury before beginning the focused history and physical examination. Rapid trauma assessment is a hands-on examination of the patient to evaluate his or her condition and should be performed after the focused history and physical examination.

136. D: During rapid trauma assessment, the head and neck should be assessed first, followed by the chest. Chest inspection should be followed by auscultation of the lungs, then palpation of the abdomen.

137. D: Because some patients attempt to control their respiratory rate during assessment, it may be necessary to count respirations to obtain a more accurate reading. After assessing the pulse, the EMT-I should keep his or her hands in place but count respirations instead. When obtaining a radial pulse, place the patient's arm across the chest, finish taking the pulse, and count respirations instead. Because some patients are abdominal breathers, chest movement is not adequate in assessing breathing.

138. C: Apnea is the absence of breathing; normal breathing is known as eupnea. Bradypnea is characterized by slow respirations and tachypnea by rapid and shallow respirations.

139. A: Pulse oximetry is unreliable in unstable patients, such as those with hypotension or hypothermia, anemia, or severe vascular disease, and in patients in cardiac arrest.

140. B: The detailed assessment is a subjective and objective examination of a patient to obtain more detailed patient information than that provided by the initial and focused assessments. In the case of priority patients, detailed assessment should be performed en route to the hospital; in the case of a patient with a life-threatening condition, immediate transport may be necessary and there may not be sufficient time to complete the detailed assessment. If a patient is not able to provide a patient history, the history may be obtained from bystanders. Elderly patients should be addressed by their formal names, such as "Mr" or "Mrs," unless the patient asks otherwise.

141. A: Unequal pupils normally occur in 2% to 4% of the population. Unequal pupils may be caused by head injury, bleeding in the brain, eye trauma, or cataract surgery; however, this condition is not indicative of drug use.

142. C: Subcutaneous emphysema is caused by air entering the subcutaneous tissue through a hole in the trachea; patients often complain of a crackling or crunching sensation below the skin. Neck vein distention may be indicative of congestive heart failure or cardiac tamponade; ecchymosis may signify neck trauma and subsequent airway obstruction. Battle's sign is a discoloration of the area behind the ear and may indicate skull fracture.

143. D: The Glasgow coma scale is used for neurologic assessment of a patient in critical condition; the maximum score is 15 and the minimum score 3. Adults scoring less than 9 have a poor prognosis. The three main areas assessed by the Glasgow coma scale are eye opening, verbal response, and motor response; 6 is the maximum score in the motor response category.

144. B: The false vocal cords or vestibular folds consist of elastic connective tissue covered by folds of mucous membranes; the false vocal cords prevent air from leaving the lungs as well as foreign materials such as liquids or food from entering the airway. The true vocal cords lie below the false vocal cords and consist of cordlike structures that vibrate to produce sound. The glottis is the slit-like opening between the vocal cords. The thyroid cartilage that comprises the main laryngeal cartilage is known as the Adam's apple.

145. C: Carbon dioxide is carried to the lungs in three ways: dissolved in plasma, combined with hemoglobin, or combined with water as carbonic acid.

146. A: A decline in oxygen saturation results in a reduction in oxygen content; thus, with 90% saturation, the partial pressure of oxygen (PO_2) falls to 60 mm Hg, with 75%, to 40 mm Hg, and with 50%, to 27 mm Hg.

147. B: Upper airway obstruction may be caused by the tongue or teeth, vomiting, swelling due to allergic reaction or smoke inhalation, and epiglottitis. Cricoid pressure is a means of preventing gastric distention or regurgitation.

148. D: The whistle-top suctioning catheter is a small, flexible tube capable of extending into the lower respiratory tract to remove fluid, blood, vomitus, and other secretions. The tonsil tip suctioning catheter is effective in removing larger particles and larger volumes of secretions and may be useful during laryngoscopy.

149. B: Procedures and devices useful in providing assisted breathing include the demand-valve resuscitator and automatic ventilator as well as mouth-to-mouth and mouth-to-mask breathing; the whistle-top suctioning catheter is used to remove fluid, blood, vomitus, or secretions from the airway.

150. C: The esophageal-tracheal Combitube should only be used in unconscious patients; it is not indicated in responsive or semiresponsive patients with a gag reflex or in those with esophageal disease.

Special Report: Difficult Clients

Every EMT-I will eventually get a difficult client on their list of responsibilities. These individuals can be mentally, physically, and emotionally combative in many different environments. Consequently, care of these persons should be conducted in a manner for personal and self-protection of the EMT-I. Some of the key guidelines are as follows:

1. Never allow yourself to be cornered in a room with an individual positioned between you and the door.
2. Don't escalate the tension with verbal bantering. Basically, don't argue with the individual.
3. Ask permission before performing any normal tasks in an individual's environment whenever possible.
4. Discuss your concerns with other people on the scene. Consult the acting supervisor if necessary, especially when safety is an issue.
5. Get help from other individuals when offering care. Get a witness if you are anticipating abuse of any kind.
6. Remove yourself from the situation if you are concerned about your personal safety at all times.
7. If attacked, defend yourself with the force necessary for self-protection and attempt to separate from the individual.
8. Don't put yourself in a position to be hurt.
9. Get the necessary help for all transfers.
10. Respect the individual's personal property.
11. Get assistance quickly, via vocal projection or the radio, if a situation becomes violent or abusive.
12. Fill out an incident report for proper documentation of the occurrence.

Special Report: Guidelines for Standard Precautions

Standard precautions are precautions taken to avoid contracting various diseases and preventing the spread of disease to those who have compromised immunity. Some of these diseases include human immunodeficiency virus (HIV), acquired immunodeficiency syndrome (AIDS), and hepatitis B (HBV). Standard precautions are needed since many diseases do not display signs or symptoms in their early stages. Standard precautions mean to treat all body fluids/ substances as if they were contaminated. These body fluids include but are not limited to the following blood, semen, vaginal secretions, breast milk, amniotic fluid, feces, urine, peritoneal fluid, synovial fluid, cerebrospinal fluid, secretions from the nasal and oral cavities, and lacrimal and sweat gland excretions. This means that standard precautions should be used with all patients.

1. A shield for the eyes and face must be used if there is a possibility of splashes from blood and body fluids.
2. If possibility of blood or body fluids being splashed on clothing, you must wear a plastic apron.
3. Gloves must be worn if you could possibly come in contact with blood or body fluids. They are also needed if you are going to touch something that may have come in contact with blood or body fluids.
4. Hands must be washed even if you were wearing gloves. Hands must be washed and gloves must be changed between patients. Wash hands with at a dime size amount of soap and warm water for about 30 seconds. Singing "Mary had a little lamb" is approximately 30 seconds.
5. Blood and body fluid spills must be cleansed and disinfected using a solution of one part bleach to 10 parts water.
6. Used needles must be separated from clean needles. Throw both the needle and the syringe away in the sharps' container. The sharps' container is made of puncture proof material.

Special precautions must be taken to dispose of biomedical waste. Biomedical waste includes but is not limited to the following: laboratory waste, pathology waste, liquid waste from suction, all sharp object, bladder catheters, chest tubes, IV tubes, and drainage containers. Biomedical waste is removed from a by trained personal.

The health care professional is legally and ethically responsible for adhering to standard precautions. They may prevent you from contracting a fatal disease or from a patient contracting a disease from you that could be deadly.

Special Report: Basic Review of Types of Fractures

A fracture is defined as a break in a bone that may sometimes involve cartilaginous structures. A fracture can be classified according to its cause or the type of break. The following definitions are used to describe breaks.

1. Traumatic fracture – break in a bone resulting from injury
2. Spontaneous fracture – break in a bone resulting from disease
3. Pathologic fracture – another name for a spontaneous fracture
4. Compound fracture – occurs when fracture bone is exposed to the outside by an opening in the skin
5. Simple fracture - occurs when a break is contained within the skin
6. Greenstick fracture - a traumatic break that is incomplete and occurs on the convex surface of the bend in the bone
7. Fissured fracture – a traumatic break that involves an incomplete longitudinal break
8. Comminuted fracture – a traumatic break that involves a complete fracture that results in several bony fragments
9. Transverse fracture – a traumatic break that is complete and occurs at a right angle to the axis of the bone
10. Oblique fracture- a traumatic break that occurs at an angle other than a right angel to the axis of the bone.
11. Spiral fracture – a traumatic break that occurs by twisting a bone with extreme force

A compound fracture is much more dangerous than a simple break. This is due to the break in skin that can allow microorganisms to infect the injured tissue. When a fracture occurs, blood vessels within the bone and its periosteum are disrupted. The periosteum, covering of fibrous connective tissue on the surface of the bone, may also be damaged or torn.

CPR Guidelines for Professional Rescuers

Topic	Adult	Child	Infant
	Past puberty	1 y/o - puberty	Under 1 y/o
Conscious Choking	abdominal thrusts (or chest thrusts in pregnant/obese)	abdominal thrusts	5 back slaps and 5 chest thrusts in infant
Unconscious Choking	Begin chest compression. Look in the victim's mouth for foreign body before giving breaths.		
Rescue Breaths Normal breath given over 1 second until chest rises.	10-12 breaths per minute (1 breath every 6-8 seconds)	12-20 breaths per minute (1 breath every 3-5 seconds)	20 breaths per minute (1 breath every 3 seconds)
Chest Compressions to Ventilation Ratios (Single Rescuer)	30:2		
Chest Compressions to Ventilation Ratios (Two Rescuer)	30:2	15:2	
Chest Compression rate	At least 100/minute		
Chest Compression Land Marking Method	two hands center of the chest, even with nipples	one hand center of the chest even with nipples	2 or 3 fingers, just below the nipple line at the center of the chest
Chest Compression Depth	At least 2" compression (hands overlapping)	about 2" compression or 1/3 the AP diameter (only heel of one hand)	about 1 ½" compression or 1/3 the AP diameter (2 fingers)
Activate Emergency Response System	As soon as you realize that the victim is unresponsive	After 5 cycles of CPR	After 5 cycles of CPR

Checklist:

- Check the scene
- Check for responsiveness – ask, "Are you OK?"
- Adult - call 911, then administer CPR
- Child/Infant – administer CPR for 5 cycles, then call 911
- Open victim's airway and check for breathing
- Two rescue breaths should be given, 1 second each, and should produce a visible chest rise
- If the air does not go in, reposition and try 2 breaths again
- Check victim's pulse – chest compressions are recommended if an infant or child has a rate less than 60 per minute with signs of poor perfusion
- Continue 30:2 ratio until victim moves, AED is brought to the scene, or professional help arrive

Online Resources

Due to our efforts to try to keep this book to a manageable length, we've created a link that will give you access to all of your online resources:

mometrix.com/resources719/emtint99

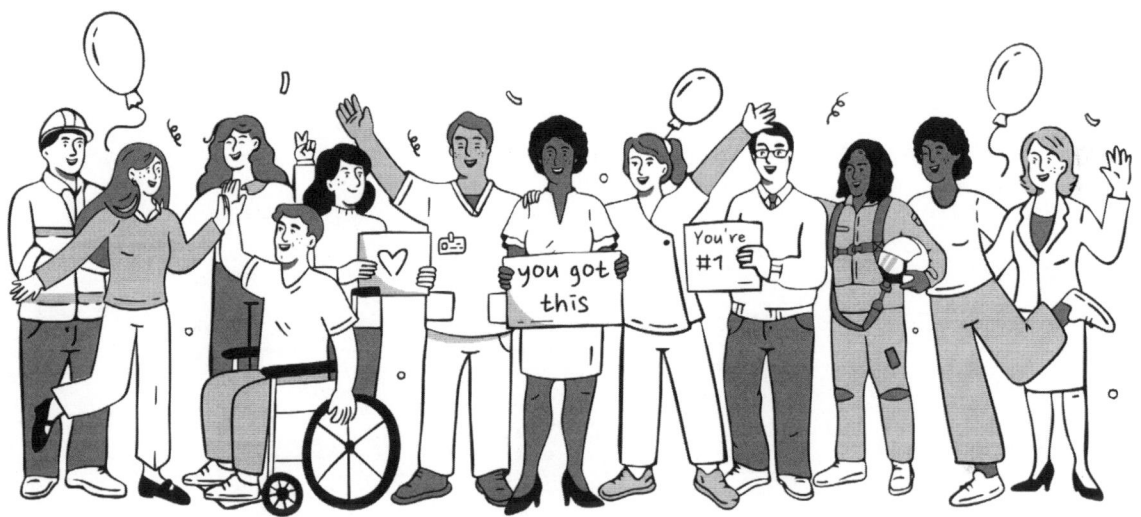